ISBN: 978-1-967-696-01-7
Published through Global Creative Group LLc

Printed in the United States of America

First Edition

www.globalcreativegroup.tech

A STEADFAST HEART: A WARRIOR'S JOURNEY THROUGH STAGE 4 OVARIAN CANCER

Contents

Forward

It is with love, respect, and appreciation that I share the beauty of the character of Glendina Greene, the author of "A Steadfast Heart." She is truly a Jewel to the Kingdom of God.

I have known Glendina since childhood and recognized the anointing on her life from our initial meeting. I met her at a church service I attended. I then noticed that she was attending conferences where I ministered. It was there that I had the opportunity to really touch spirit to spirit with her. As people would say, she had a strong anointing for such a young woman, the spirit of a seasoned woman of God or an old soul.

After several years of occasionally seeing Glendina in service, I hadn't seen her for an extended period. I learned that she was a very faithful member of a very prominent ministry in the local area. She was an adult when I saw her again, and in passing.

God truly blessed my husband and me to be a part of a ministry and be in the evangelistic field for about twenty years. My husband was then called to pastor. The transition in ministry was smooth for years, but then turbulent times came for me. During this time, Glendina visited our ministry, which was truly God-ordained. On that first occasion, the Holy Spirit quickened me to ask if God had sent her there, and she immediately responded that He had. As I walked away, the Holy Spirit prompted me to ask if He sent her there for me. She immediately responded, "Yes."

Our journey began as we began to pray together and started our intercessory prayer team. God blessed me in so many ways. I truly experienced iron sharpening iron. She had been through so much in her young life and had such great faith. What a Prophetess of God! She caused me to push forth in ministry and was with me in establishing a ministry for women and teen girls. The Word of God is used for overall covering as we educate in areas of domestic violence, health, single parenting, finances, and other regions of degradation that women and teen girls encounter. We work diligently to bring forth Chayil women – women of excellence. She continues to work with me in the ministry even with us being in different states.

The day arrived, Glendina shared that she would be moving to Atlanta. My heart was truly heavy, but I knew her intimacy and submission to God. We continued our work together in the ministry. One day, I received a call from her, and she shared that she was not feeling well. Of course, we prayed. We continued our intercessory prayer group and prayed fervently for her. After a few days, she called to say that she was in the hospital and had a series of tests done. While waiting for the results, she boldly declared the Word of God with such confidence. We bombarded heaven with her. Our decree was and is, "Fear thou not; for I am with thee be not dismayed; for I am thy God: I will strengthen thee; yea, I will help thee; yea, I will uphold thee with the right hand of my righteousness. "(Isaiah 41:10)

A Steadfast Heart A warrior's Journey Through Stage Ovarian Cancer
I shall never forget the call I received from her saying that she had been diagnosed with stage 4 ovarian cancer. I was shattered. As a spiritual mom, I had to rebound quickly and shift to decreeing what God's Word declares. She was steadily reassuring me that it was going to be okay. She said, "God is with me, First Lady." Her cheerful laugh, which is a norm for her, bursts forth. God always gives her strength for the journey. Regardless of all her experience God gives her strength to help others amid what she is going through. Because of her intimacy with God, I know a divine assignment is attached to her trial. You will be blessed by sharing and embracing her journey. A "Steadfast Heart" will bring salvation, restoration, and healing to the nations. To God be the glory!

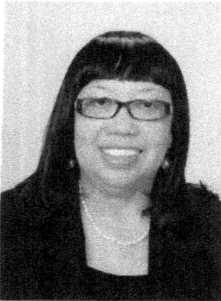

Dr. JoAnn Braziel

CEO Founder Of JB Ministry

Dedication

To my family and friends who have faced cancer, those who have passed on, and those who are thriving.

To everyone reading this book who is thriving through this disease, I stand with you.

To the phenomenal healthcare team who supported me: my doctors, surgeons, nurse navigator, social workers, hospital staff, and all who played a role in my care, thank you.

To my sisters Tiffany, Charyse, and Corlette; my church family at Mount Zion Missionary Baptist Church; my spiritual parents, Dr. Philip, and Dr. JoAnn Braziel; my mentor, Ambassador Dr. Renee Knorr; and Global Women Wealth Warriors (GW3); you all inspire me.

To everyone who supported me with monetary love gifts, kind words, and prayers, your generosity and encouragement carried me through.

This book is for you.

Introduction

When I was diagnosed with stage 4 ovarian cancer, my world transformed instantly. It was not merely a diagnosis but a call to fight, endure, and rise above one of life's most significant challenges. My journey is my steadfast faith, unwavering determination, and the profound realization that even in the darkest moments, a strength within us can shine brighter than we ever imagined.

Life is often described as a battle, with challenges and hardships acting as the battlefield. My personal journey with cancer has been one of the most intense battles I have ever faced. But as I endured the physical, emotional, and spiritual toll of this diagnosis, I made a deliberate choice: I would approach this battle as a soldier, steadfast and unmovable, determined to give purpose to what I was experiencing, no matter how hard it got.

The Bible reminds us in 2 Timothy 2:3, *"You therefore must endure hardship as a good soldier of Jesus Christ."* This scripture became my anchor, guiding me to see myself as a warrior one who does not retreat in the face of adversity but presses forward with resilience, determination, and faith. Just as a soldier trusts their commander and stays committed to the mission, I have trusted God to guide me through this process, giving me the strength to endure, persevere, and ultimately triumph.

Raising cancer awareness is not just about sharing facts, it is about empowering individuals to take proactive steps in their health journey. Understanding the signs, symptoms, and risk factors of cancer can lead to earlier detection, better treatment outcomes, and can save lives. It is vital to educate ourselves and others about the importance of regular screenings, genetic testing, and listening to our bodies. Knowledge is power, and when we arm ourselves with information, we take the first step toward preventing the devastating impact that late-stage diagnoses can bring.

Prevention and self-care go hand in hand in the fight against cancer. Prevention involves making intentional choices to safeguard our health, whether it is through a balanced diet, regular exercise, or eliminating harmful habits like smoking. But it also extends beyond the physical to include mental and emotional well-being. Stress, overwork, and neglecting our emotional health can take a toll on our bodies. Embracing self-care is a declaration that our well-being matters—that resting, nurturing our spirits, and prioritizing our needs are essential parts of living a healthy, balanced life.

To be a soldier in life's battles, one must also be steadfast. **Steadfast** means to be firmly fixed in purpose, unwavering, and resolute, even when faced with obstacles or uncertainty. This unwavering faith and resolve are beautifully expressed in **1 Corinthians 15:58**, which says, *"Therefore, my beloved brethren, be steadfast, immovable, always abounding in the work of the Lord, knowing that your labor* *is not in vain in the Lord."* This verse has reminded me that every effort, every prayer, and every act of perseverance has meaning and value in God's more excellent plan.

Central to my journey and message is the importance of being kind to oneself. Facing a diagnosis like stage 4 ovarian cancer has taught me that compassion does not only extend outward; it must also include how we treat ourselves. Kindness to oneself means letting go of guilt, silencing self-criticism, and embracing grace on even the most challenging days. It means celebrating small victories, allowing time to heal, and recognizing that we are doing our best. This mindset is not just healing—it is empowering, creating space for resilience and hope to flourish. When we combine awareness, prevention, self-care, and self-kindness, we equip ourselves to face life's battles with strength and purpose.

The title of my book, *A Steadfast Heart: A Warrior's Journey Through Stage 4 Ovarian Cancer,* reflects this mindset. It is a declaration of my choice to remain steadfast and unmovable not just surviving my journey with cancer but thriving through it by trusting in God's purpose for my life. My story is one of standing firm, abounding in faith and action, and finding strength in God's promises, even when the road seemed impossibly hard. This title is not just about my battle; it is about encouraging others to see themselves as warriors in their own lives, embracing their challenges with courage and faith.

This experience has underscored the critical importance of community. No one navigates this path alone. I am surrounded by a family and church family who enveloped me in love, a healthcare team that provided exceptional care, and a network of friends and advocates who lifted me in prayer. My unshakeable faith in God anchored me and gave me the courage to keep moving forward.

You will discover my story, practical tools, and spiritual encouragement in these pages. The *30-Day Prayer Book* and the manual *Navigate Your Cancer Journey: Staying Organized and Empowered* are separate companion resources crafted to complement this book. The prayer book offers daily spiritual nourishment, while the manual provides actionable strategies to help you stay organized and empowered throughout your treatment and recovery. Both companions are available for separate purchases and are designed to enhance and deepen your journey.

My life demonstrates hope, healing, and the power of believing that all is well when God is in the midst. This book stands as a testament to the power of steadfastness, faith, and the conviction that through love, prayer, and perseverance, we can rise more potent than ever before. It is a narrative for warriors, caregivers, and anyone seeking inspiration amidst life's most significant challenges. Through this journey, I have learned that I am never alone. Therefore, let us embrace this journey together, trusting that we will never be alone, even in the most challenging moments.

Why Decreeing and Declaring Is Important

Definition of Decree

A decree is an authoritative order or proclamation establishing something as law or truth. In the spiritual context, a decree is a statement of faith that aligns with God's Word and is spoken with authority and confidence. When we decree, we exercise the power and authority God has given us to establish His promises in our lives, declaring them truth over our circumstances.

Definition of Declare

Declaring means announcing, affirming, or speaking something openly and with conviction. In the context of faith, declaring involves boldly speaking God's Word and promises into your life. It is an act of agreement with His truth, reinforcing your faith and aligning your words with His divine plan.

Why Decreeing and Declaring Is Important

- **Aligning with God's Word**: When you decree and declare, you align your thoughts, words, and actions with God's promises. Speaking His Word aloud reinforces your belief and creates a spiritual atmosphere of faith.

- **Activating the Power of Words**: Proverbs 18:21 says, *"Death and life are in the power of the tongue."* Our words have creative power, and by speaking words of life through decrees and declarations, we release blessings, healing, and transformation into our lives.

- **Strengthening Faith**: Declaring scripture and affirmations reminds you of God's faithfulness and helps you stand firm in the face of challenges. It shifts your focus from fear or doubt to trust in His promises, helping you stay spiritually grounded.

- **Overcoming Negative Circumstances**: When life's battles seem overwhelming, decrees and declarations help you speak victory over your situation. They shift the narrative, empowering you to see your circumstances through the lens of faith rather than despair.

What This Exercise Brings About

- **Spiritual Authority:** Decreeing and declaring affirms your spiritual authority as a believer. It reminds you that through Christ, you have the power to bind and loose things on earth, as stated in Matthew 18:18.

- **Transformation of Mindset:** This practice renews your mind by replacing negative or limiting beliefs with God's truth. It cultivates a mindset of hope, courage, and possibility, helping you move forward with confidence.

- **Manifestation of God's Promises:** Speaking affirmations and scripture over your life invites God's power into your situation. As you declare His promises, you set the stage for His Word to manifest in tangible ways.

- **Encouragement and Strength:** In times of hardship, decrees and declarations provide a source of encouragement. They remind you of who God is and who you are in Him, helping you press on with renewed strength.

DIAGNOSIS

Hidden Words Within Diagnosis

God's Sign Go

So, I go.

God is Nodding Adding and Aiding

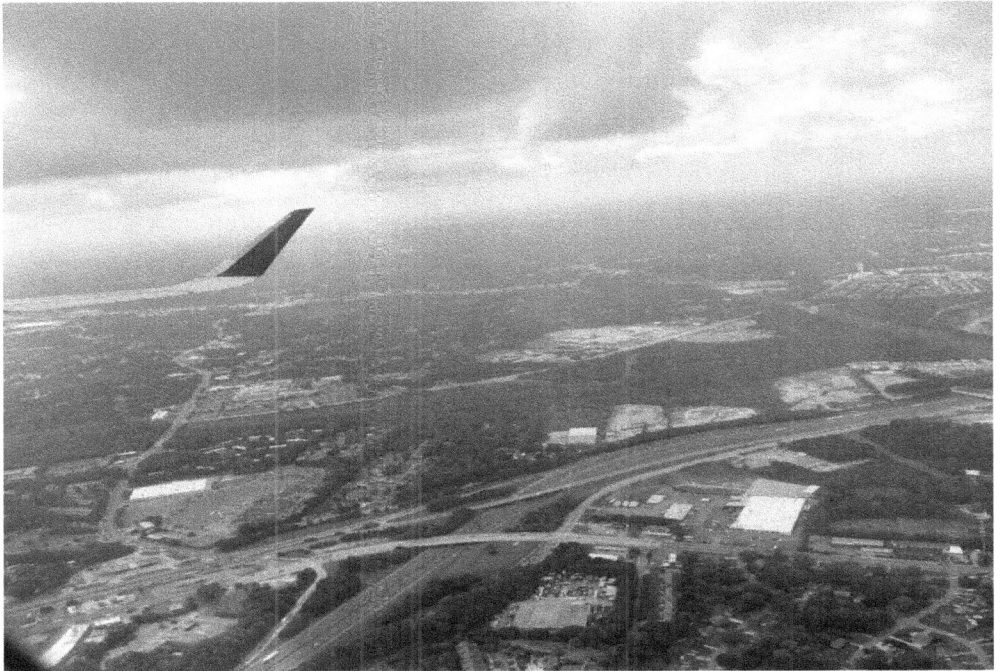

Chapter 1 The Diagnosis: Facing the Unthinkable

Psalm 37:23 The steps of a good man are ordered by the Lord: and he delighted in his way.

My journey began with a bold move to Georgia, a decision that filled me with excitement and anticipation. I was eager to meet new people and tackle the goals I had meticulously planned. Every dream, every milestone was written down, and I had an unclouded vision of how I would achieve them. The first thing I noticed about Georgia was how different the weather felt compared to West Palm Beach. The air seemed heavier with pollen, which led to me relying more on allergy medication than ever before. At times, I found myself struggling to breathe. However, this was not entirely new to me; I had experienced similar issues back in West Palm Beach, so I was not overly concerned. My mentor frequently urged me to see a doctor, but without health insurance at the time, it was not a feasible option. Just to clarify, it was not my habit to go without health coverage; there were circumstances beyond my control that made it impossible during that period. I kept hoping the problem would resolve itself.

But as time went on, more warning signs appeared, pushing me closer to seeking medical help.

I vividly remember a day when I couldn't laugh without erupting into a fit of coughing. It was uncomfortable to put it mildly. Even though this persisted, I still did not consider it a sign that something was amiss with my health. What struck me as even more unusual was my inability to speak for a long time without pausing for breath. Conversations became difficult, and there were moments on the phone when people would ask, "Are you still there?" because of my long pauses.

The final incident happened during a day of volunteer service. My coughing and shortness of breath flared up again, and my mentor asked if I needed an ambulance. Once again, I declined, convinced it was not serious enough to warrant a trip to the emergency room. A friend went to the pharmacy and picked up Tylenol and Benadryl, which offered temporary relief. It was only a matter of time before I realized something more serious was unfolding. My mentor reiterated the importance of seeing a doctor and clarified that she would not accept no for an answer. She informed me that, according to Georgia law, no one could be denied healthcare. While I was not entirely convinced, I agreed to go to the hospital. She guided me on the steps I should take upon arriving. Although I decided to seek medical attention, I was still uncertain about which day I would go.

A Steadfast Heart A warrior's Journey Through Stage Ovarian Cancer

On a quiet Sunday evening, I heard God's still, small voice urging me to go to the emergency room the following day. Early on Monday morning, May 4, 2024, around 9:00 a.m., I made my way to the hospital. I was not experiencing obvious symptoms like coughing or breathing issues at that moment. However, the moment I walked through the doors of the emergency room, I suddenly began to struggle with my breathing.

I explained my symptoms to the front desk administrator, noting that I was experiencing shortness of breath and chest pain. She recorded my information and directed me to sit while waiting for a doctor. About five minutes later, I once again heard God's still, small voice warning me that another breathing episode was imminent. Acting immediately, I alerted a staff member about my worsening condition. As I spoke, I collapsed and was quickly placed in a wheelchair and rushed into emergency care.

Though I was not fully alert, I could hear the medical team around me discussing the situation and examining my condition. The doctor identified issues with my lungs, leading to my admission to the hospital, something I had not anticipated that day.

After being stabilized, a doctor informed me that I had fluid in my lungs and that a sample would need to be drawn to determine its source. Later that day, two syringes of fluid were extracted from my lungs and sent to the lab for testing. I was taken to the radiology department for a CT scan to understand the issue better. The scan revealed over 1.5 liters of fluid in my lungs. That same day, a pulmonary specialist performed a procedure known as thoracentesis.

Before the procedure began, the attend physician asked me to sign a consent form, and the pulmonary doctor overseeing it immediately set me at ease. She was calm, composed, and reassuring, giving me a sense of confidence that everything would go smoothly. Her demeanor made all the difference in preparing me mentally for what was to come.

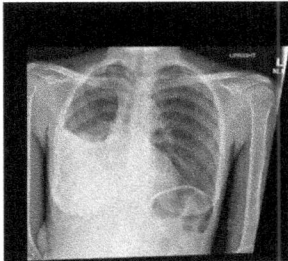

Fluid On Lung

One and a half liter of fluid in right lung.

I was positioned on a hospital bed and directed to sit in the center with my feet hanging over the side. In front of me, the medical staff placed an adjustable table, topped with a pillow to provide support. I leaned forward onto the pillow, a posture that felt a bit strange at first but made sense as the doctor explained the process.

She described each step in detail as she worked, ensuring I understood what was happening and why. First, she thoroughly sterilized the area where the catheter would be inserted. She explained that this step was crucial to prevent infection and to help keep me as still as possible during the procedure.

As the procedure began, she informed me that I might start coughing, which could feel alarming but was entirely normal. She also mentioned that while most of the fluid would be removed, it might not be completely drained. Removing only what was necessary was key to relieving symptoms while avoiding complications.

I appreciated her clear communication throughout the process, it was comforting to know what was happening at each stage. Afterward, I was even able to take a picture of the fluid that had been collected. Seeing the volume of fluid in the bag was both humbling and a moment of profound gratitude. I could not help but thank God for preserving my life through it all. The experience left me with a deeper appreciation for skilled medical professionals and the intricate procedures they perform to save lives.

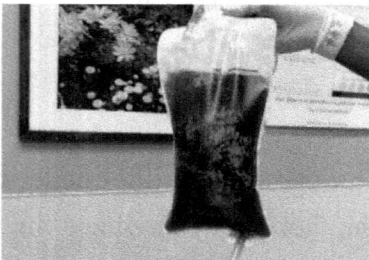

Fluid Buildup in the Lung

"Thoracentesis is a medical procedure where a needle is used to remove fluid from the lungs. wall. In this case, the fluid buildup indicated stage 4 ovarian cancer, necessitating the procedure to help alleviate symptoms and diagnose the cause."

A Steadfast Heart A warrior's Journey Through Stage Ovarian Cancer

The following morning, I lay peacefully in my hospital bed, sleeping on my back. I sensed someone entering the room, and when I opened my eyes, I saw two doctors standing quietly, waiting for me to awaken. Their patience and empathy left an impression on me that I will never forget.

It was at this time I was informed that I had stage 4 ovarian cancer. The doctors explained that the cancer had metastasized to my lungs. They also shared that the fluid in my lungs had accumulated for several months, based on its color. They informed me that my right lung had collapsed, but my left lung was compensating effectively, which explained why my oxygen saturation levels remained at 100%.

While the diagnosis was unexpected, I was not overwhelmed. The peace of God enveloped me, offering reassurance and strength in a moment that could have otherwise been devastating.

During this time, the doctor overseeing my case entered the room to deliver the news, unaware that I had already been informed. She knelt beside my bedside and expressed her desire to communicate my diagnosis personally. She assured me that she would ensure I received the help and support I needed—and she stayed true to her word. Through her efforts, I was able to secure the healthcare necessary for my journey.

As she spoke to me, I was reminded of a series of dreams I had before this moment. In the dream, I found myself in a predominantly white room. Suddenly, a small white bear entered the room.

Moments later, an enormous white bear entered the bathroom and remained there for a period of time before it left. Shortly after, a woman appeared, wearing what resembled a tan safari jacket. She stood before me and then knelt. Behind her, the large white bear reentered the room and knelt. As the woman began to speak, I heard the voice of the Holy Spirit speaking through her.

In the dream, the Holy Spirit assured me not to be afraid and prepared me for upcoming challenges, promising that all would be well. I was also told that I would receive the peace I needed throughout the experience. Additional revelations were made during this dream, which I took note of upon waking. Remarkably, I drifted in and out of this dream over the course of a night, waking up for extended periods before falling back asleep. Each time I returned to sleep, the dream resumed precisely where it had left off; this happened five times in total.

When the doctor knelt beside me in the hospital, the scene triggered vivid memories of the dream. She was wearing the same color jacket as the woman in the dream. The doctor's words conveyed that she felt lead to help me, which aligned with the Holy Spirit's message. Lastly, as I reflected on the significance of the number five in the dream, I realized that I would be discharged on Friday, the fifth day of my hospital stay. The white bear was also symbolic of having the courage and resilience to go through the journey.

After being discharged from the hospital and attending my first follow-up appointment, one of my foremost questions to my oncologist was, "What is my prognosis?" My inquiry caught my oncologist and another doctor who was in the room off guard. They exchanged glances as if surprised that I would ask such a question so soon. Their reaction suggested that many patients may not want to confront their prognosis at such an early stage.

For me, however, knowledge was power. The more I understood, the better equipped I felt to navigate challenges. My oncologist explained that prognosis is primarily influenced by early detection, which plays a critical role in cancer outcomes. Unfortunately, because I had been diagnosed with stage 4 ovarian cancer, it was too soon to provide a clear prognosis. Several factors need to be considered, including my response to treatment, overall health, and willingness to adhere to the recommended medical plan.

She then emphasized the importance of genetic testing and early detection. At that moment, she scheduled an appointment with a genetic counselor for me. She explained that individuals carrying BRCA1 or BRCA2 gene mutations should be closely monitored. In fact, as a preventive measure, women with these genetic markers are often advised to consider having their fallopian tubes removed by their 40s. Research has shown that many cases of ovarian cancer originate in the fallopian tubes, and their removal can significantly reduce the risk of developing the disease.

The conversation reinforced the importance of proactive healthcare, asking difficult questions, seeking knowledge, and making informed decisions about my future.

Healthcare Proxy

Receiving a diagnosis of stage four ovarian cancer did not feel like a death sentence; rather, it deepened my appreciation for life. Each morning, I wake up with gratitude, recognizing the opportunity to fulfill my purpose. Every individual is on this earth for a reason, and I have chosen to focus on living intentionally rather than dwelling on the inevitability of death.

I was advised that clear guidance regarding your wishes is one of the most valuable gifts you can provide your family, especially those responsible for your healthcare and financial decisions. By explicitly communicating your preferences, you relieve your loved ones of the burden of making uncertain decisions during challenging times. This is where a healthcare proxy becomes essential.

A healthcare proxy is a legal document that authorizes a trusted individual to make medical decisions on your behalf if you are unable to do so. This designated person will adhere to your expressed wishes and act in your best interest, ensuring that your values guide any critical healthcare decisions. Given the severity of my diagnosis, appointing a healthcare proxy became a crucial step in my care planning. I emphasize the importance of establishing a healthcare proxy before undergoing any life-altering treatments.

During this challenging period, Tiffany and Charyse flew into Atlanta to help prepare me for the journey ahead. We stayed together in an Airbnb, meticulously planning my future living arrangements. I would need to move from Buckhead to Union City. Moving from Buckhead to Union City was quite an adjustment. Living in the heart of Buckhead, I was surrounded by the city's fast-paced energy, high-end shopping, fine dining, and vibrant social scene. Everything was within reach, a quick ride to Midtown or a short walk to restaurants and stores. Uber rides were relatively short and affordable.

During our stay at the Airbnb, I remembered the wise words my mother had shared with me during her hospitalization. At that time, my nephew had already been born, and my sister had welcomed her second child into the world. We were all together at the hospital. Our mother took the time to advise us to cherish the time we shared together, reminding us that life is unpredictable and that we might ultimately find ourselves living in different parts of the world. My mother's words have proven to be true, and I am profoundly grateful for the moments that God allows us to be together during this time of need.

Now, in Union City, the atmosphere is quieter and suburban. It offers a sense of peace and space, and the distance from Atlanta's core is noticeable. The cost of Uber rides was extremely high when I needed to go into the city. I stayed in Union City for 3 months. During my time in Union City, I stayed in a shared house where I

A Steadfast Heart A warrior's Journey Through Stage Ovarian Cancer rented out a room and shared a bathroom with a few other people. The space was quiet, and everyone had jobs during the day. I

remember having a conversation with God where he placed it in my spirit that I would move into my own apartment before I had surgery. I stay in a place of readiness because I knew that if God said it there was no doubt it was going to come to fruition.

A Warrior's Wisdom

- Be careful not to depend only on personal knowledge.

- Seek professional help early about matters that concern you.

- Take the time to get to a quiet place so that you can listen to your body.

- Document any changes in your body.

- Build a dedicated support system of individuals and organizations you trust.

- Stay educated and up to date about your condition and treatment options.

- Ensure that all questions get answered by writing them down in advance.

- Confront your fears by seeking guidance and wisdom when uncertain.

- Be kind to yourself.

Decree and Declare this Declaration Over Your Life

1. I decree and declare, according to 1 Corinthians 6: 19-20, that my body is a temple of strength and healing.
   - **1 Corinthians 6:19-20 (NIV):** *"Do you not know that your bodies are temples of the Holy Spirit...Therefore honor God with your bodies."*

2. I decree and declare, according to Jeremiah 30:17, that my body is restored, and all my wounds are healed.
   - **Jeremiah 30:17 (NIV);** *"But I will restore you to health and heal your wounds, declares the LORD."*

3. I decree and declare according to Isaiah 40: 29 that you, Father God, give me strength and power in my time of weakness.
   - **Isaiah 40:29 (NIV):** *"He gives strength to the weary and increases the power of the weak."*

4. I decree and declare according to 2 Timothy 1:7 that I have the spirit of power, love, and soundness of mind.
   - **2 Timothy 1:7 (NKJV)** *"For God has not given us a spirit of fear, but of power and of love and of a sound mind."*

5. I decree and declare, according to Malachi 4:2, that because I fear your name, Father God, you will rise and bring healing to my mind, body, soul, and spirit.
   - **Malachi 4:2 (NLT):** *"But for you who fear my name, the Sun of Righteousness will rise with healing in his wings."*

6. I decree and declare, according to Romans 8:37, that I am more than a conqueror because God loves me.
   - **Romans 8:37 (NKJV):** *"Yet in all these things we are more than conquerors through Him who loved us."*

7. I decree and declare, according to 3 John 1:2, that I prosper in all things, that I am in good health, and that my soul is prosperous.
   - *3 John 1:2(NKJV): "Beloved, I pray that you may prosper in all things and be in health, just as your soul prospers."*

8. I decree and declare according to Isaiah 41: 10 that I am neither fearful nor dismayed because you, Father God, strengthen me and are my helper.
   - *Isaiah 41:10 (NKJV): "Fear not, for I am with you; Be not dismayed, for I am your God. I will strengthen you; yes, I will help you."*

9. I decree and declare, according to Romans 8:28, that all things are working together for my good because you love me and called me for your purpose.

   - **Romans 8:28 (NKJV)** *"And we know that all things work together for good to those who love God, to those who are the called according to His purpose."*

10. I decree and declare, according to 1 Thessalonians 5:8, that I am giving you thanks, Father God, in accordance with your will in Christ Jesus.

   - **1 Thessalonians 5:18 (NIV):** *"Give thanks in all circumstances; for this is God's will for you in Christ Jesus."*

A Prayer of Faith

Dear Heavenly Father,

I come before You wholeheartedly, asking that You heal and give me courage. In this moment of uncertainty, I choose to trust in Your unfailing love and power. You are the Great Physician, the Healer of all wounds, and the Restorer of all things.

Lord, I pray that Your peace, which surpasses all understanding, will guard my heart, mind, body, soul, and spirit. Father, I thank You for Your word stating that You have not given me a spirit of fear but of power, love, and a sound mind. I am therefore resting on that promise.

Father, I ask that you strengthen me. Thank you for giving me endurance and hope in every moment. Father, thank you for surrounding me with love, support, and wisdom. Guide the hands of the doctors and the healthcare team. Let every treatment be effective, every cell be restored, and every moment be filled with Your presence.

Lord, when the road feels long, be my refuge. When doubt creeps in, be my assurance. When my body feels weak, you are my strength. For I know that I am not alone. Thank You, Father for walking with me, fighting for me, and holding me in the palm of Your hand.

I declare healing, restoration, and victory in Jesus' name. No diagnosis is greater than Your power; no battle is more potent than Your love. May Your will be done, and may I rise from this journey with a testimony of Your faithfulness.

In Jesus' mighty name,

Amen.

Hidden Words Within The Word Chemotherapy

The Year The Hero Appears

Care, hope, empathy, meet oath, therapy, hero, ear, rare, armor, prayer, year.

Care found me.

Hope ray inside me.

Empathy inside me I choose my path wisely

Meet the new me, arm to ace my new pace.

Oath to commit with hope to cope.

Therapy creates a map, theme, team he, her, they, them pay heart art.

Hero rises inside me the heat intensity purifies me

Ear to hear peace is here.

Rare because Mother Earth therapy is here.

Armor the warrior wears: helmet, breastplate, sword, shield.

Prayer, the Path that God is there here.

YEAR THE HERO APPEARS!

Chapter 2 Enduring the Storm: My Chemotherapy Journey

"Peace, I leave with you; my peace I give you. I do not give to you as the world gives. Do not let your heart be troubled and do not be afraid." John 14:27

When I got back home, I began to reflect upon all the warning signs I may have ignored. There were two notable signs that I did not pay attention to when I was experiencing more vaginal discharge than normal. I attributed this to the aging process and thought nothing of it. I just decided to wear sanitary napkins, even though at that time, my cycle was not on. I also remember having a breakout on my abdominal area that stands all the way from my back. This breakout also triggers another condition that I was dealing with neurofibromatosis also known as NF1. The NF1 fibroids had become inflamed. This was a warning sign and something I should have paid more attention to. I am putting this information in this book and hope that readers will take all symptoms that they are experiencing and seek medical help. Leave nothing up to assuming for you can be facing a life-threatening Condition.

My First Chemotherapy Treatment

For my first chemotherapy session, my family and church family collaborated to decide who would accompany me during the process. My spiritual parents' granddaughter volunteered to stay with me for a few days. She also offered to pick me up after my treatment. She advises me to dress warmly and comfortably because she was a caregiver for her mother and knew that my first experience should be free of any unnecessary discomfort.

On the day of my first treatment, I felt well-prepared. I wore comfortable clothing as suggested. The treatment center had arranged for a driver to pick me up, and I received a call notifying me of the driver's arrival. I quickly gathered my belongings and headed outside. During the ride, I shared my diagnosis of stage 4 ovarian cancer with the driver. He responded, "I was wondering if you had cancer, those are typically the patients I transport." However, you do not look or sound like someone who was diagnosed with cancer." I thanked him for his kind words. At the time, my hair was styled in a ponytail with long single braids, and I held onto my faith, continuously reminding myself of God's promises in the Bible. I often repeated, *"All is well, and this too shall pass,"* a phrase that brought me peace in the face of challenges.

When we arrived at the cancer center, I entered through the main doors, where a security check was required. Once through security, I proceeded to the eighth floor for check-in. The receptionist greeted me warmly and said, "Ms. Green, please have a seat, and we'll call you shortly." After about 30 minutes, the treatment room doors opened, and a nurse called out my name. Upon entering, the nurse took my weight and my blood pressure. I weighed eighty-eight pounds at the time, and my blood pressure was within normal range. The nurse then escorted me to the treatment area and allowed me to choose my preferred room. I selected a room with a large window overlooking the city. Its beauty provided a calming atmosphere. The nurse asked what I would like for a snack, and I requested chips, graham crackers, apple juice, and water.

The nurse began preparing my medications, carefully laying them on the table. She reviewed each medication with me, explaining the process. One of the medications was Benadryl, which I was instructed to take orally. The rest were to be administered intravenously to ensure proper hydration and to coat my stomach in preparation for chemotherapy. The chemotherapy bag arrived covered in a brown protective wrap to shield it from sunlight. Before administering the treatment, the nurse followed protocol, reading my name and medication details aloud, which a second nurse confirmed. This procedure reassured me that the process was thorough and accurate.

Once everything was set, I called family and friends to inform them that my treatment would take approximately four hours. I told them

I would turn my phone off during the session and contact them afterward. Then, I began to pray:

Heavenly Father, I thank You that this chemotherapy will go only to the areas of my body where it is needed. I thank You that it will not damage or harm any other organs or systems in my body. Father, I thank You for Your peace, power, and protection. In Jesus' name, Amen.

After praying, I listened to praise and worship music to center myself. During my first treatment, I was visited by my social worker. I overheard her speaking with the nurse, saying she was looking for me. Upon entering the room, she introduced herself and presented me with a thoughtful gift bag from the Georgia Ovarian Cancer Alliance. Inside the bag were several items, including a purple blanket, a water bottle, an ovarian cancer teal pin, a hat, and a handwritten card with the words, *"You got this."*

The social worker explained her role to me, which brought me comfort. She said she would serve as a key support point throughout my treatment journey. Her role included connecting me with resources like support groups and financial assistance. After the social worker left the room, I finally had a quiet moment to absorb what was happening fully. Chemotherapy was now flowing through my veins. Surprisingly, I felt a deep sense of calm and peace, so much so that I drifted off to sleep during most of the session.

I was eventually awakened by the urge to use the restroom. The nurse gently reminded me of a critical safety protocol: after each use, I needed to flush the toilet three times to reduce the risk of exposing others to the chemo agents. I carefully stood up and began making my way, guiding my mobile IV pole alongside me a scene I had only witnessed in films, now made real in my own journey. Life has a way of placing us in experiences we never anticipate.

Afterward, I returned to the comfort of my recliner chair, grateful for the quiet moments of rest. I closed my eyes once more, allowing sleep to carry me through until the end of my treatment session.

I also remember that was the day the audio version of my book, *in a Cage with the Door Wide Open: Set Free* was played in the GW3 Global Society's "Praying It Forward" room on Clubhouse. Clubhouse is a social audio app that allows individuals worldwide to assemble to gather in a virtual room to engage in discussions, share motivational messages, and offer encouragement.

That day, I said a prayer, thanking God that my story of freedom from childhood abuse was being shared in a space designed to inspire and uplift others. I prayed it would reach someone who was silently suffering and bring them a sense of hope and liberation. The moment brought peace to my spirit.

The next day, I heard how my story had touched the hearts of those listening to the Praying It Forward room on Clubhouse, and I felt doubly blessed. Now, here I am again, sharing another chapter of my journey. What an incredible blessing it is to be able to share my story with those of you reading my book currently.

Walking on Ice: Reclaiming Strength Through Chemotherapy

The first time I felt the tingling in my hands and feet, I did not panic, I prayed. I had heard about neuropathy before, the way chemotherapy could sometimes affect the nerves, but I also knew something greater: nothing, not even cancer, was more significant than God. Cancer has a name, and anything with a name can be called out, confronted, and conquered. So, I spoke words of life over my body, declaring healing, strength, and peace.

During treatment, I placed gloves on my hands that had inserts for ice packs and socks with inserts as well. The cold pressed deep into my skin, numbing my fingers and toes, but I welcomed it. The ice helps prevent the chemotherapy treatment from settling into my nerves, reducing the risk of long-term damage. It was uncomfortable, but I saw it as temporary discomfort for lasting protection. Through it all, I reminded myself that this was a process, a season, and I was walking through it with faith, not fear.

Neuropathy did come, but I refused to let it steal my courage. At times, it began as a subtle itch, spreading like tiny ripples before turning into a deep, electric sensation. Other times, it felt like waves of warmth and coolness shifting beneath my skin. The pain typically began around noon, lasting into the evening and sometimes extending into the following day. But I also found relief in prayer, in resting when my body called for it, in knowing that pain was not permanent. I also called on friends and family to pray for me.

With each round of treatment, I learned to listen to my body and advocate for my needs. Finding the proper medication for nerve pain took time, and that is okay. If one thing does not work, there is always another option. I tried three different medications before finding the right fit, persistence made all the difference. My advice? Speak up. Do not settle for suffering in silence; healing comes when you ask, seek, and trust that solutions exist.

Even now, neuropathy lingers, but I no longer see it as something that holds power over me. The sensation is different now. It is more numbing, like walking on cold ice. There were days, my feet tingled as if reminding me of where I had been, and the battle I had fought. But I keep walking forward. I manage it without daily medication, only taking what I need when I need it. The key is knowing your body and doing what is best for you. Pain does not have to define you, and neither does fear.

Reclaiming Strength in the Journey

Chemotherapy is a treatment. It is a step toward healing, not something to fear. There were days when my hands felt weak, and standing for extended periods was not possible, but I adjusted. I learned to prepare meals ahead of time, to ask for help when needed, and to extend grace to myself. If there were days when I had to order food, so be it my health comes first. There is no guilt in doing what you must do to care for yourself.

This experience also deepened my awareness of my body, emotions, and thoughts. I became intentional about nourishing not just my physical health but my spiritual and mental well-being. I spoke

affirmations over myself daily, declaring that I was strong, that my body was healing, and that God's power was more significant than anything I faced. Cancer may have had its moment, but it did not write my story; I did.

One of the most important things I learned was the necessity of rest and protection. After each round of chemotherapy, I was advised to isolate for four days to allow my immune system time to rebuild. At first, the idea of isolation seemed daunting. But I reframed it as a time of renewal, a moment for my body to restore itself. My cells were replenishing, my body was working hard, and I honored that process. The truth is that chemotherapy temporarily depletes the body, but healing can follow with proper nourishment. Increasing my protein intake helped

tremendously, but everyone's body is different, so always consult your doctor to find what works best.

Staying Active and Moving Forward

Staying active, even in small ways, helped prevent complications like blood clots and kept my body strong. My regimen consisted mostly of stretching because walking and standing on my feet would trigger nerve pain. I reminded myself that even the most minor steps forward were still steps.

There is wisdom in listening to your body, but there is also wisdom in pushing just a little further than you want to go. Movement is

healing. It is a declaration that I am still here, fighting and winning even on difficult days.

Through it all, I held onto my faith. I prayed through the pain, and every time, I found relief. I spoke the Word of God over my body, declaring that healing was mine and that strength was already within me. Cancer may have a name, but God's name is more significant. Every challenge, every side effect, every problematic moment I faced them with faith, knowing that this was just a season. And seasons change.

The Importance of Self-Compassion

For much of my life, I prioritized the needs of others above my own. It was not until I found myself drained and unfulfilled that I realized the importance of self-compassion. I decided it was time to offer myself the same care, support, and dedication I had so freely given to everyone else.

I often made promises to myself, such as completing a book project or pursuing personal goals. Yet, whenever a friend or even my family called needing help, I felt compelled to put their needs first. This pattern continued for years, leaving my aspirations neglected. Repeatedly, I broke promises to myself, forcing my mind and body to endure the weight of unmet commitments.

But what happens when you consistently break your promises to yourself? What kind of message does that send to your mind and body? Over time, self-neglect can manifest as emotional fatigue, feelings of rejection, and even physical distress. Your body begins to doubt your intentions, questioning whether you will ever follow through on the commitments you made.

When you do not do the things you promised yourself, several things can happen:

- **Feelings of Disappointment or Guilt:** You might experience regret or frustration with yourself for not following through on your intentions.

- **Lowered Self-Esteem:** Repeatedly not meeting your expectations can lead to declining self-confidence and self-trust.

- **Missed Opportunities for Growth:** Each action you commit to is a chance to learn and grow. Not taking those steps might slow down your progress.

- **Revaluation of Goals:** Sometimes, failing to follow through can be a sign that you need to reassess your priorities or the feasibility of your goals, which can be a valuable learning experience.

When you do the things you promised yourself, several things can happen:

- **Satisfaction:** Experience a sense of accomplishment

- **Increase in self-esteem**: Trusting in the wisdom and abilities God has given you.

- **Embracing opportunities:** Accelerate your personal progress.

- **Affirmation of Goals:** Successfully following through can validate your priorities and the feasibility of your goals, reinforcing your commitment to them.

This realization led me to adopt a new motto: Be kind to yourself.

Now, I make it a priority to sit in stillness and truly listen to my body. In these quiet moments, I ask myself, How are you feeling today? I take the time to acknowledge any physical discomfort, assess emotional well-being, and reflect on what might be causing stress or concern. By identifying the origin of these feelings, I can take intentional steps to shift my mindset and improve my well-being. When I honor my body and mind in this way, I feel a sense of gratitude, knowing I am seen, heard, and respected. I encourage you to do the same.

Take time for self-check-ins. Ask yourself:

1. How am I feeling physically?

2. Where am I experiencing tension or discomfort?

3. How am I feeling emotionally?

4. What is bothering me, and where is that feeling rooted?

Acknowledge your emotions without judgment. Recognizing how you feel is the first step toward healing, because healing encompasses not just physical aspects. It is both emotional and mental.

As you reflect, be sure to:

- Forgive yourself for any past mistakes.

- Show yourself compassion for the times you have been too hard on yourself.

- Create peace within your mind and body by engaging in activities you can manage at this time.

- Connecting with people in healthy relationships, and embracing experiences that bring you joy, fulfillment, and happiness.

I encourage everyone to practice these principles so that you can grow intentionally, creating a path from having knowledge to applying wisdom and from information to transformation.

You deserve to live a life filled with peace, love, and contentment. Affirm this truth daily:

- **I deserve safety and security**- freedom from harm, danger, and fear in both physical and emotional environments.

- **I deserve to be happy**- to experience a deep sense of contentment, peace, and joy. Knowing that my life is in alignment with God's purpose and plan.

- **I deserve to be loved** – The right to be loved, valued, and accepted for who I am.

- **I deserve the best that life has to offer** -To have peace, love, and purpose.

- **I deserve to be heard** -Being heard involves being understood, acknowledged, and having one's opinion respected.

- **I deserve respect**- To be treated with dignity, equality, and consideration by others.

- **I deserve freedom and Autonomy**- The power to make decisions for my life without unjust control or coercion.

- **I deserve access to Health Care** – The ability to receive medical attention, preventive care, and support for mental and physical health.

- **I deserve Education and Knowledge-** The opportunity to learn, grow to my full potential, and to expand my mind and skills.

Speak this truth:

- I have peace.
- I am happy.
- I have love.
- I have the best that life has to offer.

- I have Education and Knowledge.
- I have **freedom and Autonomy.**
- I have the best care.
- I have a voice
- I have access to Health Care

I Smile

I Smile

I laugh freely!

I rest peacefully!

I love openly!

I dance gracefully!

I speak wisely!

I write knowledgeably!

I walk humbly!

I observe quietly!

I work skillfully

I Learn willingly!

I coach effectively

I empower purposefully!

Therefore, I freely, peacefully, openly, gracefully, wisely, knowledgeably, humbly, quietly, skillfully, willingly, effectively, and purposefully smile.

Ringing the Bell

Life has a remarkable way of foreshadowing our most profound moments. I recently found an Instagram post of a young woman ringing a bell, an image of triumph and emotion. She stood in what appeared to be a hospital, though my own experience tells me it was a cancer treatment center. I watched as she walked down the hallway of the cancer center; her steps spoke for itself until she reached a gleaming, gold-colored bell. With trembling hands, she rang it, and as the sound echoed, she covered her face, tears cascading down in waves of relief, victory, and perhaps even disbelief. Surrounding her were people, caregivers, supporters, and loved ones, all celebrating this hard-won milestone. At that time, she spoke no word; however, her body language said it all.

For me, ringing the Bell marked the conclusion of my final chemotherapy treatment. Ever since my diagnosis, I imagined it

would be a meticulously planned event, one I could announce to friends and family with anticipation: *"On this day, I will ring the bell." However, that was not the experience I had. Because* life, in

Its unpredictability had other plans. I was in a deep sleep when the nurse gently woke me, her words pulling me from the fog of exhaustion: *"Your treatment is complete."* She smiled warmly and asked if I would like to ring the Bell. Still sleepy, I did not respond right away. The world was still reassembling itself around me. But after 3 quiet moments, clarity returned, and with it, my answer: *"Yes."*

I had my phone and iPad with me that day, and the nurses so thoughtfully insisted on capturing the moment I would ring the Bell. One of the nurses held my iPad while I went live on Instagram so my friends and family could witness this victory in real time. The medical staff gathered around me as a dedicated support system, their faces full of joy, their presence a testament to the compassion and excellence they had shown me throughout my journey. This occasion was most certainly a win for us all.

Looking back at the video, I noticed I rang the Bell not merely once but at least five times. Every time I rang the bell; the sound of the bell could be heard by patients who were receiving treatment at that very moment. I thought about them as the sound of the Bell echoed to all that heard it, touching their soul with an unspoken declaration that another warrior had gained a stage of victory. The song playing in the background was fitting: *"Celebrate good times, come on!"* It

was more than a melody; it was an anthem. I danced that day, and so much joy filled my heart that you, Father God, were my words.

After sharing heartfelt words of gratitude with the staff, the nurse who had administered my final chemotherapy treatment presented me with a gift, a small silver bell of my own, a tangible keepsake to commemorate the moment. Every now and then, I ring that, Bell.

The Bell is a symbol that I was cancer-free. However, it holds several essential meanings. It symbolizes that I can break through.

barriers and defeat the walls of opposition and opposing forces. I was free mind, body, soul, and spirit. And with every ringing of the bell, I am reminded that victory is not just a moment; it is a mindset, a way of living.

Celebrating the End of Chemotherapy: A Testament to God's Grace

"A cheerful heart is good medicine, but a crushed spirit dries up the bones." Proverbs 17:22 (NIV).

A few days after completing my last chemotherapy session, my mentor, Ambassador Dr. Renee Knorr and Global Women Wealth Warriors (GW3), organized a celebration to honor this significant milestone, my last treatment, and the ringing of the bell. Moments like these remind us of the importance of celebrating our victories.

The celebration was hosted at Le Colonial Atlanta, a beautiful restaurant in Atlanta. My mentor arranged a Lyft to bring me too the

event, and as I arrived, she welcomed me with her signature hug. Those who know Dr. Knorr understand the power of her hugs they are filled with genuine care and love. After exchanging hugs, we walked to the restaurant's outdoor patio, where the atmosphere was perfect. The ambiance and music created the perfect setting for this momentous occasion, which I will always cherish.

The first person to greet me was Lolita Anderson, affectionately known as "the mayor" of the Global Women Wealth Warriors for her exceptional leadership skills. She gave me a heartfelt hug and spoke my name slowly and deliberately: "Glendina, it is so wonderful to see you. You look great!" As a cancer thriver, I have come to appreciate the profound meaning behind kind words, and her encouragement brought a smile to my face that evening.

Leslee Christopher, the opera singer of our group, was also there. She greeted me warmly with a smile, a hug, and congratulations. Knowing she had recently learned of my diagnosis, her heartfelt celebration of my milestone served as a testament to God's power. Her expression said it all—the "look at God" moment that fills you with gratitude.

Cynthia McNeil arrived a little later, bringing surprises and an infectious joy. Her words, "I'm so happy to be here to celebrate with you," reflected her kind spirit. Life has a beautiful way of reciprocating—when you pour love into the world, it finds its way back to you in the most meaningful ways.

Antonia Pecot, the talented psalmist of our group, also attended. She always reminds me of the unique gifts God has placed within each of us. Her words reaffirmed the importance of recognizing and cultivating my God-given talents. As the Bible teaches us in **1 Peter 4:10 (NIV)**: "Each of you should use whatever gift you have received to serve others, as faithful stewards of God's grace in its various forms." I want to encourage those of you that are reading this book to embrace and share your gifts with the world, for our talents serve as beacons of light, bringing hope and possibility to others.

Dr. Zeudiann Coleman joined the celebration despite Atlanta's notorious traffic, thank you Dr. Z for your thoughtfulness. Knowing that you took time after a long day to celebrate with me, spoke volumes about the kindhearted person that you are.

Living in the Moment

By now, I know it is evident that I am someone who treasures moments like these—celebrating life, cherishing those around me, and creating memories to reflect on later.

That night, the restaurant's food was delightful. Among the appetizers, the beet salad stood out with its sweet and tangy flavors. For dinner, I enjoyed a perfectly cooked salmon dish that was absolutely delicious and mouthwatering. Surrounded by these phenomenal leaders, I allowed myself to savor each moment, committing the experience to memory.

Thoughtful Gifts and Their Meaning

As the evening drew to a close, it was time to open gifts. Each gift had sentimental value. From a red purse and white pearl bracelet symbolizing God's provision and elegance, to a plant representing life and renewal, every gift held deep meaning.

One particularly unique gift was a stunning orchid that I now call my "Warrior's Orchid." Its colors purple, green, and teal held special significance. The teal edges, symbolic of ovarian cancer awareness, glowed radiantly in the light, reminding me of God's message: "Let your light shine." As **Matthew 5:16 (NIV)** says: "In the same way, let your light shine before others, that they may see your good deeds and glorify your Father in heaven."

The purple center symbolized royalty and echoed **1 Peter 2:9 (NIV)**: "But you are a chosen people, a royal priesthood, a holy nation, God's special possession, that you may declare the praises of him who called you out of darkness into his wonderful light."

Meanwhile, the army fatigue pattern reminded me of **2 Timothy 2:3 (NIV)**: "Endure hardship with us like a good soldier of Christ Jesus." The orchid serves as a daily reminder of life's challenges and triumphs, as well as the beauty of resilience and faith.

A New Chapter of Possibilities

The evening concluded with the symbolic blowing out of a candle—a gesture marking the close of one chapter and the beginning of another filled with miracles, signs, and wonders. It was a moment of reflection and hope, a reminder to stay open to possibilities because, as **Mark 9:23 (NIV)**states, "Everything is possible for one who believes."

That night was filled with fun, laughter, joy, because of meaningful connections. To those reading this, I encourage you to embrace life's moments and celebrate the people around you. Remember to cherish the journey and trust in the path God has set before you. Life is precious, live it fully and gratefully.

A Warrior's Wisdom

- **Diagnosis:** Educate yourself about your diagnosis, get second opinions when time allows, and get answers to your question from your medical team.

- **Treatment:** Create a well-structured plan, remain informed, and manage side effects proactively.

- **Pain:** Identify the source of the pain, the level of the pain, on a scale from 1- 10 and what is causing it. Use medications as prescribed by a healthcare physician and utilize and explore physical therapy and alternative treatments for relief.

- **Low energy:** Prioritize your rest, nutrition, and physical activity.

- **Finances:** Explore financial aid and insurance options and ask for help from your social workers and use nonprofit resources.

- **Emotions:** Acknowledge your feelings. Assess what your needs are. Seek counseling, join support groups, and express feelings through journaling art or speaking to loved ones.

- **Uncertainty:** Stay focused on the present, practice being at peace, ask questions, when possible, seek help, and have a dedicated support system.

- **Isolation:** You may need to isolate; however, stay aware of your emotional well-being. Build a dedicated support network of family, friends, and support groups.

- **Depression:** Get help, get counseling, if necessary, talk with a trusted friend or family, and most importantly, speak to your creator.

- **Anxiety:** Practicing relaxation techniques, self-care, and breathing exercises can help reduce anxiety.

- **Appetite loss:** Work with a nutritionist to find manageable, nourishing meals.

- **Side effects:** Consult doctors for symptom management, change in type of medication or dosage, and ask doctors for alternative therapy options.

- **Work struggles**: Consult employers about accommodation and rights available to you.

- **Fear of recurrence:** Practice healthy living habits, schedule follow-up appointments with your doctors, and do a mental well-being check as often as possible.

Decree and Declare this Declaration Over Your Life

1. I decree and declare, according to Philippians 4:3, that I can receive this chemotherapy treatment because you, Father God, will strengthen me through this treatment.

    - **Philippians 4:13 (NKJV)** *"I can do all things through Christ who strengthens me."*

2. I decree and declare according to Exodus 15:26 that you, Oh Lord, are the one who will heal my body; therefore, this chemotherapy treatment will bring no harm to my body, mind, soul, and spirit,

    - **Exodus 15:26 (NKJV)** *"For I am the Lord who heals you."*

3. I decree and declare according to Isaiah 40: 31 that I will wait upon you, oh Lord, to renew my strength so that I can mount up with wings like an eagle, so I can run and not get weary, and so I can walk and not faint.

- **Isaiah 40:31 (NKJV):** *"But those who wait on the Lord shall renew their strength; they shall mount up with wings like eagles, they shall run and not be weary, they shall walk and not faint."*

4. I decree and declare, according to Jeremiah 30:17, that you, oh Lord, are restoring my health and healing all my wounds.

- **Jeremiah 30:17 (NKJV)** *"For I will restore health to you and heal you of your wounds, says the Lord."*

5. I decree and declare, according to 2 Timothy 1:7, that fear, doubt, and anxiety will not be in my mind because you, oh Lord, have given me the spirit of power, love, and soundness of mind.

   - **2 Timothy 1:7 (NKJV)** *"For God has not given us a spirit of fear, but of power and of love and of a sound mind."*

6. I decree and declare according to Philippians 4:7 that I have peace that surpasses all human understanding because you, oh Lord, guard my heart and my mind.

   - **Philippians 4:7 (NKJV)** *"And the peace of God, which surpasses all understanding, will guard your hearts and minds through Christ Jesus."*

7. I decree and declare, according to Joshua 1:9, that I am strong and have courage. Therefore, I am neither afraid nor dismayed because you, oh Lord, are always with me.

   - **Joshua 1:9 (NKJV)**: *"Have I not commanded you? Be strong and of good courage; do not be afraid, nor be*

   - *dismayed, for the Lord your God is with you wherever you go."*

Prayer Of Trust

Heavenly Father,

I come before You with a heart full of trust and surrender. As I walk through this part of my journey, I ask for Your divine presence to guide and sustain me. Lord, you are my refuge and strength, a very present help in times of need. I pray for Your protection over my body as it undergoes chemotherapy. I ask that there be no side effects and allow this treatment to work according to Your will, bringing healing and restoration to every cell.

Father, I pray for the medical team responsible for my care. Grant them wisdom, precision, and compassion as they administer this treatment. Let the hands of the medical team be guided by Your divine touch. I also pray for my mind and spirit to help me to remain strong, positive, and anchored in faith. Surround me with Your peace that surpasses all understanding.

Lord, I declare that You are my healer and the source of my hope. Let Your Word fill me with comfort and strength. I place my full trust in You, knowing that Your plans for me are good, plans to give me a future and a hope. I thank You in advance for the healing and victory that is to come.

In Jesus' name, I pray.

Amen.

HAIR

Your hair may change, but your light, spirit, and beauty remain unshaken!

Chapter 3 Letting Go: The Day I Cut My Hair

Isaiah 41:10 - "So do not fear, for I am with you; do not be dismayed, for I am your God. I will strengthen you and help you; I will uphold you with my righteous right hand."

S o many emotions are tied to a person's hair especially for a woman. And even more so for a Black woman. I have often heard the saying, "A woman's hair is her crown and glory." Growing up, I did not fully understand the weight of that statement, but my journey with my hair has taught me its truth.

By the time I turned seven, I was already getting my hair permed. My mom never explained why she started perming my hair so young, but I can only assume it was to help me fit in with my peers and make my hair more "manageable." Every two months, the perming ritual would happen to tame the "new growth" that emerged, showing my natural hair texture. I remember seeing a baby picture of myself, no more than 4 months old, with a full afro. It was beautiful, although I didn't have the words to appreciate it at the time.

Growing up, I heard people say phrases like, "Oh, you have good hair," or "You're blessed with good genes to have such beautiful hair." Within my community, hair like mine was often described as "coarse" or "nappy, "words that carried a negative undertone, as if

My naturally textured hair was not enough. These words stuck with me, shaping my view of my hair and, by extension, myself. Society placed so much value on straight, flowing hair that I internalized the idea that my natural hair was not beautiful.

When natural hair started trending, and the culture began to embrace Black women wearing their hair naturally, I started to rethink my relationship with my hair. For about two years, I wore my hair naturally, without perms or chemical alterations. But even then, I relied on sew-in weaves and wigs to create the image I thought I needed. The idea of cutting my hair was not an easy one. It felt like cutting my hair would strip me of my femininity. I have a small frame, little curves, and a petite stature. My hair was the one part of me that I felt truly connected to my femininity and letting it go felt like I was losing a piece of my identity.

Still, life had other plans. When the time came to cut my hair, it was not something I was emotionally ready to do. But I knew I had to. When you go through chemotherapy, the doctors explain to you that the regimen chosen for you, which causes hair loss, is difficult to hear. For me, the process was both physically and emotionally draining. I learned that it is better to cut your hair before the treatment begins because losing your hair can cause inflammation and tenderness in your scalp. Knowing what type of chemotherapy you are taking is crucial. If you are on a regimen that causes hair loss, cutting your hair beforehand can help prevent unnecessary pain.

After not being able to endure the pain, I was feeling from my hair falling out I remember calling my mentor, someone I deeply trusted

and admired, and asking for help finding someone who could cut my hair with care and understanding." She recommended the perfect person, Roni, who had experience in cutting the hair of women with cancer. This phenomenal woman came to my home, offering me the privacy and compassion I needed for such a vulnerable moment. She was patient and gentle, knowing how tender my scalp was. She talked to me through the entire process, as she cut away what felt like layers of my past.

The moment Roni had finished cutting, I felt my breathing change. I had to sit for a few minutes as my entire body began to realign. It was a moment of me being kind to myself. The weight I was carrying, stemming from my reluctance to cut my hair, was lifted the moment Roni cut off all my hair. My hair had held so much of my fears and insecurities. I felt a newfound sense of liberation with it gone. I did not just cut my hair; I released myself from years of expectations and societal standards. It is an experience. I will never forget. From that moment on, I never regretted it. Later that day, I remember crying tears of joy. A smile now comes to my face every time I think of that day. Therefore, I now embrace the freedom and the new level of self-awareness that comes with it.

Black hair has always been more than just hair. It is history, culture, and identity. Over the years, we have created a lexicon to celebrate and describe the beauty of our hair. Terms like "kinky," "coil," "curly," and "textured" have replaced the derogatory labels of the past. We now speak of "4C curls," "twist-outs," "protective styles," and "afros" with pride. Names like "locs," "Bantu knots," and

"Cornrows" honor the cultural roots of our hair traditions. And movements

The Natural Hair Movement has reclaimed phrases like "Black Girl Magic" and "Crown" to celebrate the beauty and resilience of Black hair.

I have adopted a new mantra: 'I will be kind to myself." I remind myself to be the friend I have been to so many others. I tell myself that God knew exactly what He was doing when He made me. I remind myself that I am an overcomer and that I can do all things through Christ, who strengthens me. I have learned to see the beauty in the image I see in the mirror every day, regardless of the season I am in.

Cutting my hair was more than just a physical act, it was a declaration of self-love and self-acceptance. It allowed me to redefine my beauty on my own terms. I hope that by sharing my story, I can encourage others to embrace themselves fully, with or without hair.

It is time we rewrite the narrative about what makes someone beautiful. True beauty lies in seeing the beauty in every human being as they are. When we celebrate our diversity, whether it is through hair or any other part of who we are, we build healthier communities, families, and friendships.

The human image is beautiful the way it is. Declare these words over your life. I released myself from all negative thoughts, behaviors, patterns, and attitudes I have embraced in the past. I now open myself up to this new me. Therefore, I embrace the freedom to love and accept who I am entirely.

A Warrior's Wisdom

- Let this be the season you try something new.

- Use this as an opportunity to celebrate your strength.

- Let your inner beauty shine.

- Be creative with wigs and head scarves.

- Walk with confidence.

- Remember that you are resilient.

- Smile, laugh, rejoice.

- Impact those around you with your story.

- Discover earrings that bring out your beauty.

- Speak words of life over yourself daily.

Decree and Declare this Declaration Over Your Life

1. I decree and declare according to Psalm 139:14 that I am fearfully and wonderfully made.
   - **Psalm 139:14:** "I praise you because I am fearfully and wonderfully made; your works are wonderful; I know that full well."

2. I decree and declare God power lives inside me.
   - **2 Corinthians 12:9:** "But he said to me, 'My grace is sufficient for you, for my power is made perfect in weakness.' Therefore, I will boast all the more gladly about my weaknesses, so that Christ's power may rest on me."

3. I decree and declare I am God handiwork.
Ephesians 2:10: "For we are God's handiwork, created in Christ Jesus to do good works, which God prepared in advance for us to do."

4. I decree and declare according to Jeremiah 1:5 that God know who I am.
Jeremiah 1:5: "Before I formed you in the womb I knew you, before you were born, I set you apart; I appointed you as a prophet to the nations."

5. I decree and declare according to 1 Corinthians 12:18 that God created every part of me the way he wanted to.

1 Corinthians 12:18: "But in fact God has placed the parts in the body, every one of them, just as he wanted them to be."

6. **I Decree and declare according to Proverb 31:30 that it is you oh God. that I fear.**

Proverb 31:30 " Charm is deceptive, and beauty is fleeting, but a woman who fears the Lord is to be praised."

7. I decree and declare I am beautiful.

Song of Solomon 4:7: "You are altogether beautiful, my darling; there is no flaw in you."

Prayer of Embracing Uniqueness and Identity

Heavenly Father,

I come before You with gratitude and humility, thanking You for the gift of life and the unique person You created me to be. Father God, I thank you that Your Word says I am fearfully and wonderfully made, and I rejoice in the beauty of Your design. Lord, I declare that I am unique, set apart by You for a purpose. Father, I ask that you help me to walk confidently in the truth of who I am, embracing every aspect of my being.

Father, I am enough because Your grace is sufficient for me. Teach me to find my worth not in the world's standards but in Your unfailing love and purpose for my life. I make the confession that I am fearfully and wonderfully made, crafted by Your hands with intention and care. I embrace that I am an original, a masterpiece in Your eyes, knowing that nobody else is like me.

I thank you, Father, for fully embracing my uniqueness and originality. I thank you that I am walking boldly in my identity. I thank you, Father, that I love myself as You love me, and I see myself through Your eyes. I release every negative thought, behavior, pattern, and attitude and embrace who You created me to be. Today, I open my heart to the new me, the me You have designed and empowered. I stand on the truth that You formed me with intention and love. Let this prayer strengthen my spirit, renew my mind, and draw me closer to Your will.

In Jesus' name, I pray.

Amen.

GENETIC TESTING

"Knowing your story's blueprint,

empowers you to shape your destiny with knowledge and courage."

Glendina Green

Chapter 4 Uncovering My Roots: The Importance of Genetic Testing

"But I will restore you to health and heal your wounds,' declares the Lord." Jeremiah 30:17

From the moment I received my diagnosis, I made a promise to myself: I would document my journey and share my story not just for myself, but for my family, friends, and anyone who might benefit from understanding the importance of knowing their family health history. This commitment has grown into a mission to break the silence that often surrounds hereditary conditions, equipping others with the tools to take control of their health and their future.

The Importance of Knowing Your Family Health History

Growing up, I was vaguely aware that more than ten people in my family had cancer, but the conversations were fleeting and nonexistent. It was not until I began researching my maternal family history that I uncovered the true prevalence of cancer within my family. My grandmother and several other relatives had cancer, yet no one had openly discussed it. This realization became a turning point for me. It highlighted the critical importance of genetic testing not just for myself, but to educate and share this information with my family and, eventually, with readers of the book I am writing.

For years, cancer in my family was concealed, or it may have been that I was not privy to certain information due to my age. There were no discussions about genetic testing or awareness of hereditary risks, such as the BRCA1 or BRCA2 mutations. Many family members, including myself, were blindsided by diagnoses, unprepared for the realities of our shared history. This lack of awareness highlights the importance of breaking the cycle of silence. Understanding genetic risks and engaging in open conversations about our health can make a profound difference not just in treating cancer, but in preventing it altogether.

Breaking the Cycle of Silence: Generational Knowledge, Not Curses

In some families, cancer is referred to as a "generational curse" due to its hereditary factor. There are those who believe it is a punishment from God for immoral behavior or disobedience for not following biblical principles. While this perspective is common, I believe it stems from a lack of knowledge and communication. We cannot break these cycles without educating ourselves and future generations as to the root cause of cancer. In my own family, silence about cancer meant no one knew to ask questions, seek genetic testing, or take proactive steps. Even survivors often did not share their experiences, leaving others in the family unprepared to face the possibility of being diagnosed with this disease called cancer.

While I respect that cancer is a deeply personal and often traumatic journey, I have learned that seeing cancer in the family may be a signal of a genetic component, like the BRCA1 mutation. This knowledge is not just personal; it is powerful. It provides an opportunity for family members to get tested, take preventative measures, and detect cancer early, when it is most treatable. Prevention and early detection are not only helpful but also lifesaving.

My Family Health Assignment

Before my appointment with a genetic counselor could be scheduled, I was asked to compile a detailed family medical history. This assignment asked for a list of family members diagnosed with cancer, including their type of cancer, age at diagnosis, survival status, and date of death if applicable. For living relatives, I noted whether they were still battling cancer or in remission. This process was a revelation. It forced me to confront how widespread cancer was in my family and clarified the importance of genetic testing for myself and others.

My Genetic Counseling Experience

The day of my genetic counseling appointment finally arrived. I brought the family history I had painstakingly compiled. The counselor reviewed my information, explained the

The significance of genetic testing and prepared me for what I might learn. A blood sample was collected that day to analyze my genes for mutations associated with cancer risk.

The counselor emphasized that genetic testing is not just about my own health. It also provides critical insights for my family. By understanding whether I carried mutations such as BRCA1 or BRCA2, I could take proactive steps to reduce my risk while helping my family understand their own potential risks. That conversation cemented my resolve to share what I learned with my loved ones and encourage them to seek testing.

Genetic Insights:

Understanding the BRCA1 and Neurofibromatosis (NF1) Mutations

My genetic test results revealed mutations in two critical genes: BRCA1 and NF1. These findings carry profound implications for my health and my family, offering both challenges and opportunities for proactive management and personalized care.

- The BRCA1 Mutation: This mutation increases the risk of breast and ovarian cancer by disrupting the gene's ability to repair DNA damage. It is inherited in an autosomal dominant manner, meaning inheriting just one altered copy of the gene from either parent is enough to increase cancer risk. My BRCA1 mutation result was inherited by my mother's side of the family.

- The NF1 Mutation: This mutation causes neurofibromatosis type 1 (NF1), an inherited condition that can lead to tumors,

- skin changes, and other complications. Like BRCA1, NF1 mutations are also autosomal dominant. If I decide to have children, research has noted that my children would have a 50% chance of inheriting NF2. The positive results of NF1 were no surprise to me because I was diagnosed at the age of twelve. However, the diagnosis of NF1 was not properly documented in my medical record. Therefore, having the genetic test done confirmed that I had NF1.

Why This Information Matters

These findings are more than a diagnosis they are a roadmap for prevention, early intervention, and better outcomes. For the BRCA1 mutation, I now have the knowledge to take proactive steps, like enhanced screenings, preventive surgeries, or lifestyle changes, to reduce my cancer risk. For the NF1 mutation, I can prioritize regular monitoring to manage symptoms and address complications early.

But the significance of these results extends beyond me. They provide a call to action for my family. Documenting and sharing this information empower my loved ones to understand their risks, seek genetic testing, and take proactive steps to protect their health.

Risk Factors for developing Cancer:

1. **Genetic Factors**: Genetic factors can cause a person to be at an elevated risk for developing cancer because of inherited mutations.
2. **Lifestyle Choices**: Lifestyle choices such as smoking, lack of proper nutrients, failure to exercise, and elevated levels of alcohol consumption.
3. **Environmental Exposures**: exposure to carcinogens can cause cancer. Types of carcinogens that can cause cancer are asbestos, UV radiation, and chemicals.
4. **Infections**: It is important to note that viruses and bacteria can also cause cancer. Here are a few examples: HPV, Hepatitis B and C, and Helicobacter pylori.
5. **Age**: Genetic damage due to the aging process can lead to cancer for some people.
6. **Random Mutations**: Changes in genetics can also cause cancer.

A Call to Action: Breaking Silence, Saving Lives

As I reflect on my journey with cancer, I am reminded through each experience that knowledge is power. If cancer has touched your family, I urge you to take the time to gather your family's health history. Ask the challenging questions. Encourage open conversations. Take steps to understand whether genetic risks may be present. Early detection and prevention are not just possibilities; they are opportunities to save lives.

A Steadfast Heart A warrior's Journey Through Stage Ovarian Cancer

Together, through education, compassion, and action, we can break the silence, fight fear, and create a legacy of health and empowerment for future generations. Let us turn genetic risk into a proactive plan for a healthier tomorrow.

Decree and Declare this Declaration Over Your Life

1. I decree and declare, according to James 1:5, that I now ask
   you for Wisdom on how to navigate this journey, and I thank
   you for your generosity in answering this request. That "
   - James 1:5 NIV: "If any of you lacks wisdom, you should
     ask God, who gives generously to all without finding fault,
     and it will be given to you."

2. I decree and declare, according to Isaiah 26: 3 NIV, that my
   mind is steadfast because I put my trust in you. I that you,
   Father, that I now have perfect peace because of this truth.
   - Isaiah 26:3 NIV: "You will keep in perfect peace those
     whose minds are steadfast because they trust in you."

3. According to Philippians 4:13 NIV, I decree and declare that I
   can handle the results of this genetic test because You
   strengthen me.
   - Philippians 4:13 NIV says, "I can do all this through him
     who gives me strength."

4. I decree and declare according to Proverbs 3:5- 6 that I will
   trust in you in every challenge I have in life with my hold

heart. I thank you, Father, for helping not to trust in my understanding. Father, I submit to You this genetic test and everything that concerns me.

- Proverbs 3:5-6 NIV: "Trust in the LORD with all your heart and lean not on your own understanding; in all your ways submit to him, and he will make your paths straight."

5. I decree and declare that I am strong and courageous because You, oh God, are with me.
   - (Joshua 1:9 NIV): "Have I not commanded you? Be strong and courageous. Do not be afraid; do not be discouraged, for the LORD your God will be with you wherever you go."
6. I decree and declare according to 2 Thessalonians 3:3 NIV that you, oh God, are my strength. I thank You for your protection. I thank You for increasing my faith in Your word.

- Thessalonians 3:3 NIV: "But the Lord is faithful, and he will strengthen you and protect you from the evil one."

7. I decree and declare, according to Deuteronomy 31:8 NIV, that You, Oh God, have gone before me to make my way clear and will be with me in everything that I do. Therefore, I walk in the great assurance that You, Oh God, are faithful, and I now walk with courage based on what You have revealed to me in Your written word.

- (Deuteronomy 31:8 NIV) "The LORD himself goes before you and will be with you; he will never leave you nor forsake you. Do not be afraid; do not be discouraged."

8. I decree and declare according to Psalm 119:105 NIV that Your word, oh God, Light my path that I may know the way to go and the decision I will need to make related to my care.
   - Psalm 119:105 NIV: "Your word is a lamp for my feet, a light on my path."

9. I decree and declare, according to Romans 8:28, that no matter what the results of the genetic testing are, Father, you will use it for good.
   - Romans 8:28 NIV: "And we know that in all things God works for the good of those who love him, who have been called according to his purpose."

10. I decree and declare that I am restored and healed through the mighty power of God working in me.
    - Jeremiah 30:17 NIV: "But I will restore you to health and heal your wounds, declares the Lord."

A Prayer of Understanding

Heavenly Father,

I come before You in humble prayer, Father. I thank you for seeking your guidance and comfort as I navigate the realm of genetic testing. Father, I thank You for fashioning me uniquely and wonderfully, and in this modern age of science, I ask that Your wisdom and love guide me in understanding the marvels of our creation.

Your Word reminds us in Psalm 139:13-14, "For you created my inmost being you knit me together in my mother's womb. I praise you God because I am fearfully and wonderfully made because your hands are upon me. Father, I hold fast to this truth, knowing that every genetic detail is a testament to Your divine creation.

Lord, as I learn more about my genetic makeup, help me to trust Your perfect plan for my life. Father, I thank you for Jeremiah 1:5, which states, "Before I formed you in the womb I knew you, before you were born, I set you apart." Father, thank you for strengthening my heart to accept the gift of life in all its complexity and grant me the courage to face whatever situation that may come with grace and humility.

Father, I thank you for the knowledge I gained through genetic testing, which will help me to understand my physical makeup. May the things I discover bring me closer to You, deepening my gratitude for the intricate design of my body and the precious lives You have entrusted to me.

In every cell, every strand of DNA, I see Your fingerprint. Guide the hands and minds of those working in laboratories and clinics so that their discoveries may lead to healing, hope, and a better understanding of Your wondrous creation. I ask that You bless the work of medical science and genetics with integrity and compassion. Thank You, Lord, for the gift of life and the blessing of discovery.

In Jesus' name, I pray,

Amen.

SURGERY

When we identify the enemy called cancer, we place a bullseye on it, recognizing we are not the target. With the precision of a sniper, ready aim and fire.

Yes, Urge, Sure Surge

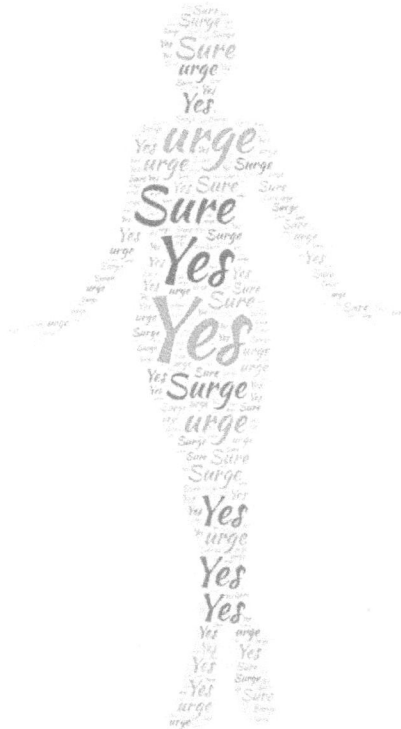

Chapter 5 The Battle Within: Preparing for Surgery

"No, in all these things we are more than conquerors through him who loved us." Romans 8:27

A t the start of this journey, I must express my immense gratitude for having the best oncologist. From the moment she delivered the diagnosis to the day we discussed surgery, her calm confidence gave me hope. She thoroughly explained the purpose of the surgery, what to expect during the procedure and the importance of my six-week recovery period. She even emphasized how vital it was to have someone to assist me upon discharge. Her detailed care and unwavering support reassured me that I was in the best hands possible.

Pre-Surgical Preparations

A hospital wristband was given to me a week before the procedure. To the hospital staff, it was a way to identify me; to me, it was a reminder of what lay ahead. Along with it came clear instructions to stop all supplements and avoid any medications that might interfere with surgery.

The date was set September 26, 2024. The night before, I was given sterile wipes and asked to thoroughly cleanse my body. "Stay indoors until you leave for the hospital," the nurse had said. It felt like a peculiar request, but I followed it to the letter, savoring the strange peace that filled the day. There was no room for fear in my heart; instead, I felt an overwhelming calm, as though I were being held in God's divine hands. I prayed, packed my essentials phone, charger, and photo ID, and called for an Uber early the following day. As the car moved through the quiet streets, I embraced the serenity that surrounded me, knowing I was prepared for whatever lay ahead.

At the Hospital

The hospital buzzed with an energy that felt safe, peaceful, and reassuring, reflecting the personal significance of my surgery. I followed every instruction using the sterile surgical cloth one last time before the nurses inserted IV lines into my arm. "We may need to place additional ports," one of them said, her voice kind but matter of fact.

Then I met the anesthesiologist. With a calm that mirrored the atmosphere, she explained what to expect. "You'll be under general anesthesia, which means you won't feel anything during the surgery," she said. "We'll monitor your heart rate, breathing, and vital signs closely to ensure everything stays stable." The medical

The team assisting the surgeon visited me before the procedure to reassure me that everything would go well and to address any questions I may have. Their presence and words further eased my mind.

I had assigned my sister Charyse as the person who would receive direct updates about my progress. The hospital had a wonderful system that allowed her to receive text messages about the progress of my surgery. She flew in that morning, but her plane landed after my surgery had already begun. Despite this, I had absolute confidence in the medical staff, knowing they would keep my sister informed every step of the way.

The Surgery

The Doctor and the medical team worked tirelessly, removing my uterus, ovaries, fallopian tubes, appendix, and the lining of my stomach, the peritoneum, to address the spread of cancer. The open surgery allowed them to thoroughly examine and debulk the affected areas, ensuring no trace of the disease remained.

When the doctor informed my sister that all the tumors in my body were nonviable and required surgical removal, it served as a significant testament to effective medical intervention and positive outcomes. So many people had been lifting me up in faith, and hearing that report answered every one of those prayers. Charyse later told me how the surgeon's compassionate and thorough explanation left her in awe. She could not wait to share the miraculous news with our family and friends.

Waking Up

Coming out of anesthesia felt like stepping into a dream that was slowly fading away. A distant voice called out my name, Ms. Green, and as I blinked my eyes open, I could only see a figure standing before me, the world gradually coming into focus. While I felt some discomfort in my abdomen, the nurse's soothing words provided reassurance: "You are doing great." Shortly after, members of the surgical team visited to check on me and confirm that the surgery had gone well. Their kindness and calm demeanor were comforting.

I was in the recovery area, where I remained for observation until a room became available. Once settled into my room, I suddenly felt the urge to use the restroom and pressed the call button for assistance. To my surprise, the nurse informed me that I had a urinary catheter. It served as a reminder of the importance of being aware of the changes in my body. At that moment, I began to check myself for any other changes I was not yet aware of, realizing just how crucial it is to remain conscious of my physical well-being.

A dietitian then entered the room and inquired about my food preferences. Following a pescatarian diet, I shared that I mostly enjoyed fruits, vegetables, and fish. She politely informed me that I would need to include more protein and carbohydrates in my diet to recover. At the time, I had already placed my food order for the day. When my meal arrived, I noticed that the order had been altered. I asked the dietary aide about the change, and she explained that the dietitian had modified my meal plan for the remainder of my hospital stay. While I did not get exactly what I wanted, I appreciated the adjustment, understanding that sometimes what I need is more important than what I desire.

I only need the urinary catheter on the day of the surgery and one day after that. The next day would involve a physician therapist coming in to ensure that I start walking again on my own without assistance. My recovery went well; my primary oncologist came in to visit to explain how the surgery went and to provide me with information about the stitches and how I was to take care of them. "We've used absorbable stitches," she explained. "They'll dissolve naturally as your body heals, so you won't have to worry about having them removed." She outlined the steps for recovery, including no heavy lifting for six weeks, plenty of rest, and careful attention to the incision to prevent infection. It was also at that time that she did an assessment of my abdomen to ensure that everything was going as planned. One of the questions asked was whether I was passing flatus, in other words, if I was passing gas. My answer was yes; however, although I was passing gas, I was not having a bowel movement. It is noted that having surgery and being under anesthesia and pain medication can cause postoperative ileus. Which means it can stop the normal intestinal flow. I often hear the doctors say that my bowels were still waking up. Noting that before I could be released from the hospital that I needed to have a bowel movement.

My sister Charyse stayed in a nearby hotel and visited me daily. She made sure I was comfortable and eating well (though I could have done better on that front). Her presence brought me so much comfort. The joy and relief in her voice when she shared the good news with others were contagious. We both recognized how blessed I was to be surrounded by a community of prayers and unwavering faith. Tiffany and Charyse flew into Atlanta to ensure that I was confirmable for the journey ahead. The three of us stayed together at an Airbnb and planned the details related to my chemotherapy treatment and living arrangements. I had to move out of Atlanta for a few months until a financial plan could be put in place. Remember praying to God that by the time I had my surgery, I would be in my new place.

At that time, I remembered the words of my mother during her time in the hospital, my nephew was already born, and my sister had a second child on the way. We were all at the hospital with our mother, and she told us to cherish the time we had together. She stated that you never know where life can take you, and you all may end up living in different parts of the world. Tiffany was we are going to College in Gainesville, and I was currently living with Charyse. Now that the statement that our mother made had come to pass, we were all living in different places. So, I most certainly thank God for the times he allows us to come together.

Mrs. Antonia Pecot also visited me at the hospital, bringing gifts. We share a common love for the Lord and the color green. She gifted me a green cream-colored mug that quoted Matthew 19:26 With God, all things are possible. A notebook that quoted the words Jeremiah 29:11" I know the plans I have for you declares the Lord plans to prosper you and not to harm you, plans to give you hope &

a future." I love the scripture, so these words resonated with my spirit. I recall that healing is possible with God, regardless of its form. Yes, God could have healed me without having to go through chemotherapy or without having to have surgery; however, healing can come in many forms. He allows the tools of chemotherapy and surgery to help aid in the healing process. God has placed doctors in place as part of the healing process. He uses his words to bring me comfort and to let me know that he always has a plan, no matter what life circumstances bring my way. The key for me is to trust God in the process. I can now join in with my heavenly father and declare that I will experience prosperity, and I have hope for the journey that awaits me. There is no fear living inside of me because I understand God's plan for my life. Not only do I understand that God has a plan, but I also know that He places people and doctors in my life so that I can make wise choices regarding my health.

Fear arises in times of uncertainty; however, now that I understand his plan, fear has no place in my heart. I learn how to rest in the promises of God.

The Road to Recovery

Charyse stayed until Sunday, and her compassion and encouragement provided a solid foundation for my healing journey. My oldest sister, Tiffany, arrived a few days after Charyse left, stepping into her role as the eldest sibling with grace and diligence. She arrive in Atlanta on Tuesday, the day I was discharged from the hospital, and we both stayed at a nearby hotel for convenience.

During this time, I was mindful of the instructions given by my medical team. Until I could immerse my incision area in water, I performed sponge baths to maintain hygiene without risking infection. Additionally, I carefully followed the specific guidance on turning on my side when sitting up or getting out of bed. This involved bending my knees slightly, rolling onto my side, and using my arms to push myself upright. These movements minimized strain and helped me avoid injury during the critical preliminary stages of recovery.

Our time together was a precious gift. I rarely have the opportunity to spend extended time with Tiffany, who lives overseas. Each morning, we tuned in to a prayer and discussion group on the Clubhouse app in the Praying It Forward room (GW3 Global Society), where I served as a moderator. Tiffany had never heard of it before, but she was intrigued by the voices of people around the world offering prayers, sharing wisdom, and discussing faith, finance, and motivational messages. While she never spoke during the sessions, her thoughts afterward were insightful and encouraging.

Those moments became part of our healing routine. After the sessions, we would discuss my recovery and the steps I needed to take to rebuild my strength. Tiffany reminded me to rest, take small walks, and nurture my spirit. It felt like old times, like sisters catching up after being apart for years. Her presence brought comfort, and her wisdom added depth to my journey toward healing.

Reflections

Looking back at the journey feels surreal and empowering. From the time I met my oncologist I shared with my sisters, every step was a testament to faith, love, and resilience. Each consent form I signed, each prayer whispered on my behalf, and each morning spent with Tiffany in quiet reflection led me here to a place of peace and strength.

This experience taught me that peace can prevail even in the face of immense challenges. Surrounded by love, faith, and skilled hands, I navigated a season that could have been marked by fear and uncertainty, but was instead filled with hope and grace. Though the road ahead is still one of healing, I am here, standing twelve feet tall as my mentor would say, ready to embrace each new day with gratitude and joy.

Before Surgery:

1. **Educate Yourself About the Procedure:** Ensure you understand what your surgery involves. Educating yourself about your surgery will prevent guessing.
2. **Prepare Your Body:** Eat healthy meals, drink adequate water days before your surgery, and rest as much as before surgery.
3. **Create a Support System**: Ensure you have a support system to get you to the hospital and back home after your stay.
4. **Manage Medications and Allergies**: To avoid complications, know what medications you are allergic to

   and provide that information to your healthcare team in advance.

5. **Ask About Pre-Surgery Guidelines**: Your doctor may ask you to stop eating or drinking a certain number of hours before surgery or to stop certain medications. Follow these instructions carefully to prevent delays or complications.

After Surgery:

1. **Follow Post-Op Instructions Carefully**: Post-op instructions can involve wound care, pain management, and limitations on activity.
2. **Listen to Your Body**: Healing is different for everyone, so your body heals at its own time. Please pay attention to the systems you are experiencing and write them down.
3. **Pain Management:** Use prescribed pain medications as directed rather than waiting until the pain becomes severe. Staying ahead of discomfort allows for better rest and mobility.
4. **Movement:** Consult with your doctor about when you can start moving. Movement helps prevent blood clots and promotes circulation.
5. **Manage Mental and Emotional Health:** Cancer surgery can affect your physical and emotional well-being; therefore, sharing your thoughts with someone you trust becomes essential.

Know Your Options in Advance

It is crucial to be prepared for the possibility of needing a blood transfusion or Plasma. It is essential that you are ready to ask questions so that nothing will take you by surprise.

A Blood Transfusion is:

- A medical procedure where red blood cells or whole blood cells are given to patients through an IV.

- Blood transfusions are given to patients to restore oxygen levels or replace blood loss during surgery.

Plasma Transfusion is:

- Plasma is the clear liquid part of your blood that contains essential proteins and clotting factors.

- **Plasma transfusions** are given to patients to help treat bleeding or clotting issues during or after surgery.

Can A patient choose to be given a Blood transfusion or Plasma?

Yes and No It Depends:

- Patients can choose if they want to be given a blood transfusion or a plasma transfusion in nonemergency cases.

- The patient can ask the doctor for alternatives to blood transfusion.

- There are situations where the patient can choose based on their religious beliefs, comfort, or values.

- Consulting with your doctor and asking the right questions can help with the process.

No, Not Always

- Doctors are trained to act quickly in emergencies to help save a patient's life and restore balance to the body.

- When a patient's blood oxygen is low, a blood transfusion is needed for the collection of oxygenated red blood cells.

- Certain conditions require a specific product:

    - **Inadequate oxygen?** You will need a blood transfusion with red blood cells.

    - **Uncontrolled bleeding?** A plasma transfusion may be necessary.

Question to ask your healthcare team:

- What are my transfusion options?

- What are the risk factors for having a blood transfusion or plasma transfusion?

- What are the benefits of a blood transfusion or a plasma transfusion?

- Can I try an alternative first?

- What is the urgent of this decision?

Blood Transfusion and Plasma Transfusion Alternatives:

- Iron supplements or injections: Iron supplements or injections can be used instead of a blood transfusion for patients with anemia.

- Cell salvage: Cell salvage is a process that involves using a person's blood.

- Erythropoietin: Erythropoietin can be used because it helps with the production of red blood cells.

- IV fluids (volume expanders): IV fluids can be used to stabilize circulation.

- Clotting medications: Clotting medications can be used to reduce bleeding.

It is essential to note that most alternative lists, such as erythropoietin, are time-sensitive. Erythropoietin can take weeks to produce and may not be the best alternative in emergencies. The information provided is intended to inform you about what is available, aiding in making informed decisions when discussing your options with a healthcare provider.

A Steadfast Heart A warrior's Journey Through Stage Ovarian Cancer

Medical Disclaimer

This book is written from the heart of a cancer survivor who advocates for cancer prevention. The information in this book is, therefore, my personal journey with stage 4 ovarian cancer, experiences with treatment, and research I found meaningful along the way. I hope these words bring comfort, clarity, and strength to others navigating their own health challenges.

I am not a licensed medical professional. This book is not intended to diagnose, treat, cure, or prevent any disease. It should not replace the advice of your doctor or medical team. Every person's situation is unique, and what worked or helped me may not be right for someone else. Consult with your healthcare provider when making medical decisions about surgery, blood transfusions, or treatment options.

Your health is essential. Your voice needs to be heard, so speak. Your questions need to be answered, so ask. Be an advocate for yourself to ensure your decisions are implemented and your voice is respected.

Decree and Declare this Declaration Over Your Life

1. I decree and declare, according to Deuteronomy 31:8, that You, Oh God, go before and with me in the surgical room.
   - **Deuteronomy 31:8**: *"And the Lord, He is the one who goes before you. He will be with you; He will not leave you nor forsake you; do not fear nor be dismayed."*

2. I decree and declare, according to Psalm 91, that your angels have charge over me and will keep me as I go through surgery.
   - **Psalm 91:11**: *"For He shall give His angels charge over you, to keep you in all your ways."*

3. I decree and declare that my surgery will be a part of my healing process and that I will have an abundance of peace as I walk in this truth.
   - **Jeremiah 33:6**: *"Behold, I will bring it health and healing; I will heal them and reveal to them the abundance of peace and truth."*

4. I decree and declare according to Isaiah 53:5 that you on God, were wounded for my transgressions and bruised for

A Steadfast Heart A warrior's Journey Through Stage Ovarian Cancer
my iniquities and that the chastisement of my peace you bore; I
am healed because of this truth.

- **Isaiah 53:5** – *"But He was wounded for our transgressions, He was bruised for our iniquities; the chastisement for our peace was upon Him, and by His stripes we are healed."*

5. I declare that fear has no power over me because the Lord is holding my hand, calming all anxiety.
   - **Isaiah 41:13**: *"For I, the Lord your God, will hold your right hand, saying to you, 'Fear not, I will help you.'"*

6. I decree and declare strength and peace over my family and loved ones as they support me during this procedure.
   - **Isaiah 26:3** *"You will keep him in perfect peace, whose mind is stayed on You, because he trusts in You."*

7. I decree and declare that I have the peace of God that surpasses all understanding. I thank You, God, for guarding my heart.
   - **Philippians 4:7:** *"And the peace of God, which surpasses all understanding, will guard your hearts and minds through Christ Jesus."*

8. I decree and declare according to Psalm 30:2 that when I cry out to you, oh Lord, You will hear me and heal me.

   - **Psalm 30:2**: *"Oh Lord my God, I cried out to You, and You healed me."*

9. I decree and declare that I will not fear having surgery because I put my trust in You, Father God.

   - **Psalm 56:3-4** *"Whenever I am afraid, I will trust in You. In God, I will praise His word. In God, I have put my trust in him; I will not fear."*

10. I decree and declare that I will live during this surgery and declare your works, oh God, in my life.

    - **Psalm 118:17**: *"I shall not die, but live, and declare the works of the Lord.*

A Prayer of Peace in The Mist of Surgery

Heavenly Father,

Father God, I come to You as I undergo surgery. In Isaiah 41:10, You remind us, "Fear not, for I am with you," and in Psalm 23:4, Father, I thank You for comforting me with Your guidance. Father, I thank you for that.

Lord, I cling to Your promise in Jeremiah 29:11 that You have plans of hope for me, so I confess that all is well with me. In Philippians 4:6-7, You assure me that Your peace, which surpasses all understanding, will guard my heart. So, Father, I thank you for protecting my heart.

Father, I trust you completely, as Proverbs 3:5-6 instructs. In Matthew 11:28, You invite the weary to find rest in You; in John 14:27, You bestow upon me peace. Father, I thank you that I find rest in you.

You are my refuge, as Psalm 46:1 proclaims, and Your grace is sufficient, as declared in 2 Corinthians 12:9. Father, I thank you that you are my refuge, my safe place. Father, thank you for your grace, which is sufficient for me. I receive your grace.

 Finally, I hold onto Romans 8:28, trusting that You work all things together for my good.

In Jesus' name, I pray,

Amen.

Hidden Words Within the Words SUPPORT SYSTEM

The Words "Super" and "Upper" can be found in the Word Support System.

Adjectives for super: excellence, outstanding, of the highest quality, larger, greater, and more powerful than usual.

Adjective for upper: is situated above, higher in position, of a higher rank or status, located towards the top of something.

The hidden message within the words' support system' is that humanity becomes great, excellent, powerful, and of the highest quality, gaining a high-ranking status when we find the ability to support one another.

Thank you, Father God, For My Support System

Chapter 6 Support System

"Praise be to the God and Father of our Lord Jesus Christ, the Father of compassion and the God of all comfort, who comforts us in all our troubles."

2 Corinthians 1:3-4

Facing cancer is overwhelming on many levels, but one of the most significant challenges can be the financial hardship that comes with it. During this time, you often find yourself relying on the support of others to help meet basic needs, whether it is food, living expenses, or medical bills. It is important to have a support system in place I wish I had the strength to do more to meet my needs. However, that was not possible at that time. I had to show myself compassion. In those vulnerable moments, I discovered the power of leaning on family, friends, community, and organizations that genuinely care.

I want to start by acknowledging that while many believe insurance is available for everyone, whether it is life insurance, health insurance, or other financial resources, which is not always the case.

The reality is that these opportunities are not accessible to everyone. And that is okay. If you have access to them, I encourage you to utilize these resources to the fullest. Speak with financial advisors in every area of your life to help minimize the financial strain that can come with medical bills, food, and living expenses. If life insurance is available to you, it can certainly be an asset, offering peace of mind during an otherwise uncertain time.

However, even if those options are not within reach, I want you to know that help is available. I received information from the nurse navigator, who was a part of my healthcare team; she provided me with the financial assistance I needed then.

I received support from organizations like the American Cancer Society and the National Coalition for Ovarian Cancer. Both were incredible. The application process was quick, taking less than 30 minutes for each. For the American Cancer Society, I received a call from an agent who was eager to help. After gathering the basic information, I was sent a gift card via email, which I could use almost immediately. The National Coalition for Ovarian Cancer was equally effective. They asked me questions over the phone, and I received a gift card in the mail within ten business days. Their kindness left me speechless.

My church family also stepped in with rental assistance for several months. Their support was overwhelming and deeply appreciated. They came together, pooled resources, and helped cover my rent more than I could have ever asked for. I created a GoFundMe account that was a blessing. There are those who may hesitate to participate in crowdfunding, but life has a way of humbling us. You never know where you might find yourself; there is no shame in seeking help when needed. Yes, there are always stories of people misusing systems, but I focus on the good, the genuine acts of kindness from people who want to help. Every gift, regardless of its size, carries meaning. As the scripture says, *"Whoever sows bountifully will also reap bountifully"* (2 Corinthians 9:6). Every seed that has been sown into my life, whether financial, a kind word, or a simple prayer, has been a blessing beyond measure.

To those who gave anonymously, thank you. Your generosity did not go unnoticed. To my sisters, cousins, nieces, and nephews who have poured into my life in ways I cannot fully put into words. I am eternally grateful. My medical bills were manageable because of my medical team, who went beyond to ensure I got the help I needed. If you are reading this, thank you for your acts of kindness; they are truly appreciated.

As I reflect on my journey, I realize that not everyone has had the same opportunities I have, and that thought humbles me even more. Gratitude has been my constant companion through it all. Yes, there were hard days, but the financial blessings and support I received made it impossible not to say, "Thank You, God." When asked how I felt at every appointment, my answer was simple: "Great. Blessed." And I meant it. Not that every day was easy but because I was surrounded by people who cared. I was experiencing miracles daily that came without measures.

The Battleground of The Emergency Room

When telling this part of my story, I wanted to liken my visits to the emergency room to a battleground where the patients are the warriors fighting disease and enduring pain and uncertainty, while doctors, nurses, and hospital staff serve as overworked and often overstressed frontline responders. The medical professionals work tirelessly, caught in an unrelenting cycle of urgency and care. Police officers maintain order by addressing issues as they arise, bringing a sense of security. Family members, in turn, serve as advocates, ensuring their loved ones receive the care they need.

I share this story from the perspective of a warrior. As I lay on my hospital bed, the cries of fellow warriors echoed through the room, some in agony from their wounds, others pleading to go home against medical advice. Despite efforts to block out the noise, the small, overcrowded space made it impossible not to hear. A nearby patient, determined to leave, was informed by the doctor that they needed treatment. Yet, he was allowed to go home after signing a waiver acknowledging their decision. It was a reminder that we all have the right to choose the care we receive, even if it is not in our best interest.

It would be my second trip to the emergency room in less than 24 hours. After being discharged from the hospital, I received a call from a nurse urging me to return. Now, I lay against the cold wall of my hospital bed, waiting for answers. The doctor approached and explained that surgery might be necessary. A surgical team would review my case and determine the best course of action. As I waited, I updated my family and friends, bracing myself for what was to come. Half an hour later, the results came in: no surgery was needed. I would be discharged once again from the hospital and sent home.

Before leaving the emergency room that day, I lay there in that hospital bed, taking a moment to observe my surroundings. In all its chaos, the emergency room functioned as an unrelenting machine. Warriors lined the walls, waiting for care. Doctors and nurses darted between patients, consulting charts, speaking with patients, listening to patients, and listening to the family members of those patients. Nurses administer treatment as instructed by the doctor. The phrase 'excuse me' becomes a common expression as patients are placed in their designated spots on the wall, where their assigned number is displayed. The air was thick with movement; there was no such thing as stillness, no quiet moment. Even the break room, a designated space for rest, was strategically placed with an open window, allowing medical staff to watch the activity outside.

The Reality of Our Emergency Rooms

The emergency room is a paradox. On good days, medical staff are hailed as heroes; on bad days, they are merely seen as workers fulfilling a duty. But healthcare professionals are humans prone to exhaustion, stress, and mistakes. They have taken an oath to do no harm, yet the system itself often makes that promise challenging to uphold.

So, how do we fix this battleground?

1. **Increase Healthcare Staffing** – We need more hospitals, doctors, nurses, and trained medical staff. The demand for emergency care is overwhelming, and without sufficient personnel, burnout is inevitable.

2. **Improve Training and Education** – Ensuring that medical professionals remain competent and compliant is crucial. Continuous learning, skills training, and honest self-assessment of knowledge gaps should be encouraged.

3. **Address Staff Well-Being** – Healthcare workers must be in tune with their emotions. Recognizing stress and knowing when to take breaks is essential for clear thinking and optimal patient care.

4. **Encourage Patient Advocacy** – Warriors, speak up. If something feels wrong, ask questions. Holding medical professionals accountable is necessary, but so is open communication. Doctors and hospital staff are human, too, and sometimes, they need reminders when attention is required in a specific area.

5. **Create a Culture of Awareness and Compassion**

   Awareness is key. A system cannot be fixed if its flaws are ignored. Compassion must extend to everyone involved: the patients, their families, and the medical teams working tirelessly to save lives.

Words cannot express my appreciation to the healthcare team for the exceptional care, empathy, and expertise you have shown me during my journey. To my doctors, surgeons, social workers, nurses, nurse navigators, and every member of my healthcare team, thank you for your commitment and for treating me with kindness, patience, and respect.

In each of you, I experienced God's absolute best. Your unwavering support, attentive listening, and gentle encouragement have made all the difference. I am forever thankful for the blessing of having such an excellent group of people by my side during this challenging time.

Thank you from the bottom of my heart for everything you have done for me. May you be abundantly blessed in your lives for your invaluable work.

To healthcare workers, I also say this: Take the time to check in with yourself. Make the necessary adjustments to perform at your best. A clear mind allows for better decision-making, improved patient care, and fewer mistakes. Seeking guidance from colleagues when uncertain and remembering that no one should bear the burden alone.

To the warriors, I say this: Advocate for yourself. Ask questions. Voice your concerns. Extending an olive branch when needed because while

A Steadfast Heart A warrior's Journey Through Stage Ovarian Cancer doctors and nurses hold power in the system, they are also just people trying to navigate an incredibly demanding and complex field.

Yes, accountability is crucial. Malpractice must never be ignored. But real change begins with awareness, honesty, and a shared commitment to improving the system for everyone involved. The emergency room will always be a battleground, but with the right approach, we can make it a place where warriors and healers can work together to fight the good fight

A Warrior's Wisdom

1. **Give thanks:** Give thanks to God the creator of all things.

2. **Practice gratitude:** Make a list of all the people that help you throughout your journey and write them a thank you note.

3. **Wisdom:** ask God for wisdom.

4. **Trust:** Build your ability to trust others in your time of need.

5. **Positivity:** Use your journey to bring awareness and Education,

6. **Kindness:** Be kind to yourself and others.

7. **Forgiveness:** Forgive yourself and others.

8. **Impact:** Find a way to impact those around you.

9. **Support group:** Consider joining a support group for individuals living with cancer, especially one tailored to your specific type of cancer.

10. **Hobby:** Find a hobby that interests you

Decree and Declare this Declaration Over Your Life

1. I decree and declare, according to Ecclesiastes 4:9-10 that my destiny helps surround me wherever I go. I thank you, Father, for helping me when I fall, and I help them when they fall.
   - ***Ecclesiastes 4:9-10 NIV:*** *"Two are better than one, because they have a good return for their labor: If either of them falls down, one can help the other up."*

2. I decree and declare, according to Galatians 6:2, that you, oh God, are surrounding me with individuals who are trustworthy, individuals who will love me, individuals that I can support, and individuals who will support me.
   - **Galatians 6:2 NIV):** *"Carry each other's burdens, and in this way, you will fulfill the law of Christ."*

3. I decree and declare that I walk in unity with my support system according to Psalm 133:1 NIV.
   - ***Psalm 133:1 NIV:*** *How good and pleasant it is when God's people live together in unity!"*

4. I decree and declare according to Proverbs 15 22 NIV that wise counsel surrounds me.

- **Proverbs 15:22 NIV:** *"Plans fail for lack of counsel, but with many advisers they succeed."*

5. I decree and declare, according to Proverbs 27:17, that you, oh God, surround me with individuals that will sharpen me with wisdom as I sharpen them with wisdom.

   - **Proverbs 27:17 NIV:** *"As iron sharpens iron, so one person sharpens another."*

6. I decree and declare, according to 1 Thessalonians 5:11, that my support system is a source of strength and encouragement.

   - **1 Thessalonians 5:11 NIV:** *"Therefore encourage one another and build each other up, just as in fact you are doing."*

7. I decree and declare, according to 1 Peter 4:8, that I am surrounded by unconditional love and support.

   - **1 Peter 4:8 NIV:** *"Above all, love each other deeply, because love covers over a multitude of sins."*

8. I decree and declare, according to Ecclesiastes 4:12, that you, oh God, connected me with relationships of unity and

teamwork that cannot be broken. That serves as a source of strength.

- **Ecclesiastes 4:12 NIV:** *"Though one may be overpowered, two can defend themselves. A cord of three strands is not quickly broken."*

9. I decree and declare that God will bring forth individuals who speak life, wisdom, and encouragement into my spirit and circumstances.

- **(Proverbs 15:4 NIV):** *"The soothing tongue is a tree of life, but a perverse tongue crushes the spirit."*

10. I decree and declare, according to your word in James 1:17, that the gifts of family, friends, organizations, and healthcare team come from you, Father God, and I thank you for blessing me with supportive relationships.

- **James 1:17 NIV:** *"Every good and perfect gift is from above, coming down from the Father of the heavenly lights, who does not change like shifting shadows."*

Driven for Fulfillment: Is a call to fulfillment my Purpose and a Call to Action.

As I step boldly into the new season in my life, my heart beats with a singular, unwavering theme: *Driven for Fulfillment.* Driven for Fulfillment is not merely a phrase; it is a declaration of what I intend to pursue, an invisible banner to the natural eye under which I march, and a compass that guides my every thought, words, and action.

Primarily, I identify as a Kingdom representative—a believer in my Lord and Savior, Jesus Christ. It is my privilege and mission to share the good news of the Gospel, for the most significant message the world could ever receive is the message of *love.* The Bible proclaims, *"Beloved, let us love one another, for love is of God, and everyone who loves is born of God and knows God. Whoever does not love does not know God, for God is love."* This bible message is found in 1 John 4:7-8 and is the anthem of my heart: *Beloved, let us love one another.* Love remains the most radical, transformative force in the world.

I am also a social change advocate, convinced that we must not conform to environments that tolerate injustice, inequality, or complacency. We must courageously define what is ethically sound and morally right because what is acceptable to one person may not be considered acceptable to others. We must be clear in these definitions to build societies where peace and health flourish.

We cannot afford to be mediocre or desensitized to the suffering around us. It is said that one person has the power to change the world. Therefore, I decree that I will transform the community, the nation, and the global by doing my part. I am so happy for the opportunity to make an impact on those around me by telling my story and inspiring others.

After navigating the profound journey of being diagnosed with stage four ovarian cancer in May 2025, I have become a fierce advocate for cancer prevention and health awareness. My body is a sacred vessel, and caring for it is a personal responsibility and a holy act. I will be kind to myself. Knowing your family's medical history, scheduling regular health care checkups, and seeking support when needed are critical steps in being kind to oneself.

I say this to those facing health challenges: *Do not walk alone.* If fear or financial barriers hold you back, seek help. Ask boldly for help from your community, trusted friends, and, most importantly, God. When you ask, He will answer. Doors will open, and people will appear, often in unexpected forms. Sometimes, we miss the help God sends because it does not arrive in the packaging we anticipated. But trust this: when you ask God for wisdom and guidance, He will send the resources, the support, and the strength you need.

In a world that can seem desensitized to the needs of others, I challenge you to open your heart. Give when and how you can. Your reward is not in earthly recognition but in the eternal echoes of your kindness. What you do in secret, God will reward you openly. We are His hands and feet on this earth. If you have ever prayed, *"God, use me,"* then be ready to respond when the call comes to help the widow, uplift the orphan, feed the hungry, and comfort the broken.

Giving is not always monetary. Sometimes, it is a kind word, a heartfelt prayer, a smile, or simply your presence. However, you can give, *give.*

Today, I declare I will fulfill my God-ordained purpose on this earth. I proclaim that God is the driving force behind every endeavor I undertake. It is His Spirit that leads and guides me on how I am to help others, His wisdom that strengthens me, and His love that fuels me.

You, too, can make this declaration. Speak words of life over your destiny. Seek God's guidance to discover who He has called you to be and what He has appointed you to do. Let this be the season you are driven for Fulfillment not just in personal achievements but in purpose, love, and the transformative power of intentional action.

I Live to

*I live to **I**lluminate.*

*I live to **W**rite.*

*I live to **I**gnite.*

*I live to **L**ove.*

*I live to **L**ight.*

*I live to **S**peak.*

*I live to **H**eighten.*

*I live to **I**ntegrate*

*I live to **N**avigate.*

*I live to **E**levate.*

Therefore, I will illuminate, write, ignite, love, light;
speak, heighten, integrate navigate, elevate.

I will shine.

Matthew 5:16 KJ V

16 *Let your light so shine before men, that they may see your good works, and glorify your Father who is in Heaven.*

Prayer of Gratitude and Blessing

Heavenly Father,

With a heart overflowing with gratitude, I come before You today, thanking You for the countless ways You have shown up in my life through the hands and hearts of others. Thank You for every person who has sown a seed of kindness, whether through financial gifts, words of encouragement, prayers, or simply showing up when I needed them most.

Lord, I pray those facing financial hardship during their battles with illness. May You surround them with people whose hearts are open and willing to help. Bless the families, friends, communities, and organizations that step in as vessels of Your love and provision.

I pray that You bless every person who has given, whether large or small, openly, or anonymously. Let their generosity return to them in ways they never imagined pressed down, shaken together, and running over (Luke 6:38). May the lives of those who give to others be filled with abundance, joy, and peace.

Father, I pray for financial wisdom to be released over those reading this prayer. Guide them to the right resources and advisors who will help them navigate their journey with clarity and confidence. Strengthen their hearts, renew their hope, and remind them that with You, all things are possible (Matthew 19:26).

Send angels, both human and angelic forms, to meet every need. May Your grace overflow in their lives, and may they recognize Your hand in every blessing that comes their way.

In Jesus' name, I pray,

Amen.

United States National Cancer Resources

National Cancer Institute

Part of the National Institutes of Health (NIH), the NCI is the federal government's principal agency for cancer research and training. The NIH offers information on cancer types, prevention, treatment, clinical trials, and research funding.

- **Website:** Comprehensive Cancer Information - NCI
- **Contact: 1-800-4-CANCER (1-800-422-6237)**

American Cancer Society

The American Cancer Society is a nationwide nonprofit organization that eradicates cancer through research, education, advocacy, and patient support. The ACS website provides comprehensive information on various cancer types, treatment options, and support services.

- **Website:** Information and Resources about Cancer: Breast, Colon, Lung, Prostate, Skin | American Cancer Society
- **Contact: 1-800-227-2345**

Centers for Disease Control and Prevention

The CDC provides data, statistics, and cancer prevention and control information. The CDC provides resources for understanding cancer risks, early detection, and prevention strategies.

- **Website:** Cancer | Cancer | CDC
- **Contact:1-800-232-4636**

National Comprehensive Cancer Network (NCCN)

An alliance of leading cancer centers that publishes clinical practice guidelines and provides resources to help patients and healthcare professionals navigate cancer treatment.

- **Website:** National Comprehensive Cancer Network - Home
- **Contact:215-690-0300**

Cancer Support Community

The Cancer Support Community is a nonprofit organization that provides free support, education, and hope for cancer patients. They offer counseling services, support groups, and a variety of educational resources.

- **Website:** www.cancersupportcommunity.org
- **Contact:1-888-793-9355**

Susan G. Komen® for the Cure

The Susan G. Komen for the Cure specializes in breast cancer research, advocacy, and support.

- **Website:** Breast Cancer Foundation | Susan G. Komen®
- **Contact:1-877-465-6636**

National Ovarian Cancer Coalition

The National Ovarian Cancer Coalition (NOCC) is a nonprofit organization dedicated to raising awareness, providing education, and supporting survivors and families affected by ovarian cancer. It promotes early detection and advocates for improved research to enhance the quality of life for those impacted by the disease.

- **Website:** We are the National Ovarian Cancer Coalition Home PAGE - ovarian.org
- **Contact:1-888-682-7426**

Appendix A – The Acrostanza Poetic Form

Created by Glendina Green (2025)

Official Literary Definition Entry

Term: Acrostanza

Part of Speech: noun

Pronunciation: /ə-ˈkrɒ-stæn-zə/

Definition:

An Acrostanza is a modern poetic form in which the first letter of the final word in each stanza or repeated phrase forms a hidden message or affirmation when read sequentially. The form often uses repetition of a guiding phrase (e.g., "I live to…") to unify rhythm and intention, while the final words encode a second layer of meaning. (Green, 2025)

The Acrostanza Form

The Acrostanza transforms repetition into revelation. Each stanza or line begins with a repeated clause that declares purpose, while the terminal words encode an affirmation through their first letters. The poem becomes both declaration and design structure and spirit intertwined.

Form Rules

1. Select a repeated phrase (e.g., "I live to," "I choose to," "I rise to").

2. Determine a hidden message or affirmation (e.g., I WILL SHINE).

3. End each stanza with a word beginning with the next letter of that message.

4. Optionally close with a reflective statement that reveals the entire phrase.

Example (from "I Live To")

I live to Illuminate.

I live to Write.

I live to Ignite.

I live to Love.

I live to Light.

I live to Speak.

I live to Heighten.

I live to Integrate.

I live to Navigate.

I live to Elevate.

Therefore, I will illuminate, write, ignite, love, light, speak, heighten, integrate, navigate, elevate.

Hidden Message: I WILL SHINE

Appendix B – The Chemotherapy Word-Weave Poem

The Chemotherapy Word-Weave Poem

Created by Glendina Green (2025)

Definition:

A Chemotherapy Word-Weave Poem is a literary form that reveals hidden words embedded within a single, powerful source word. Each stanza or line begins with one letter from that word, forming an acrostic pattern, while simultaneously incorporating words that can be literally found within the source word's letters.

This poetic form symbolizes how healing and hope can be discovered within hardship, that even within the word "chemotherapy," one can find care, empathy, therapy, prayer, and heroism.

Structure Guidelines:

• Source Word: The base word determines the structure (e.g., chemotherapy = 13 stanzas).

• Acrostic Formation: Each stanza begins with one of the letters in sequence.

• Hidden Word Inclusion: Each line must use words that can be formed from letters in the base word.

A Steadfast Heart A warrior's Journey Through Stage Ovarian Cancer

• Thematic Purpose: Reflects transformation, courage, and divine renewal found within adversity.

• Title: The poem may include a subtitle that embodies its message of revelation or healing.

Example Poem (Excerpt)

Hidden Words Within The Word Chemotherapy

The Year The Hero Appears

by Glendina Green

Care, hope, empathy, meet oath, therapy, hero, ear, rare, armor, prayer, year.

Care found me.

Hope ray inside me.

Empathy inside me, I choose my path wisely.

Meet the new me, arm to ace my new pace.

Oath to commit with hope to cope.

Therapy creates a map theme, team, he, her, they, them, pay, heart, art.

Hero rises inside me; the heat intensity purifies me.

Ear to hear peace is here.

Rare because Mother Earth therapy is here.

Armor the warrior wears: helmet, breastplate, sword, shield.

Prayer the path that God is there here.

YEAR THE HERO APPEARS!

Symbolism:

Each word within chemotherapy becomes a revelation a message of faith woven from letters that once represented fear. The poem transforms what was once a medical term into a sacred declaration of restoration.

Appendix C The Declaration Poetic Form

Term: **The Declaration Poem**

Part of Speech: noun

Pronunciation: /ˌdek-lə-ˈreɪ-ʃən ˈpoʊ-əm/

Definition:

A Declaration Poem is a modern free-verse poetic form originated by Glendina Green (2025) that centers on affirmative, first-person statements of action and being. Each line begins with the word "I" followed by a verb and adverb expressing intentional living, peace, healing, or empowerment. The poem concludes with a reflective synthesis that transforms these actions into embodied qualities, symbolizing the journey from doing to becoming.

Structure:
• **Each line begins with "I [verb] [adverb or phrase]!"**
• **Concludes with a final sentence transforming actions into attributes.**
• **Tone: affirmative, faith-filled, and transformational.**
• **Theme: identity, healing, purpose, and joy.**

A Steadfast Heart A warrior's Journey Through Stage Ovarian Cancer

Example Excerpt (from "I Smile," Glendina Green, 2025):

I smile.

I laugh freely!

I rest peacefully!

I love openly!

I dance gracefully!

I speak wisely!

I write knowledgeably!

I walk humbly!

I observe quietly!

I work skillfully!

I learn willingly!

I coach effectively!

I empower purposefully!

Therefore, I freely, peacefully, openly, gracefully, wisely, knowledgeably, humbly, quietly, skillfully, willingly, effectively, and purposefully smile.

Appendix D – The Difference Between an Affirmation and a Declaration

Introduction

The Declaration Poem represents more than literary expression; it is a spiritual act of transformation. While traditional I Am Affirmations focus on identity and belief, Declarations bring that identity to life through action. The difference is a subtle yet profound one; one speaks of being, the other of becoming.

1. Linguistic Difference

An affirmation states who you are:

"I am strong." "I am healed." "I am worthy."

A declaration demonstrates how you live that truth:

"I stand strong." "I walk healed." "I love openly."

Affirmations describe identity. Declarations activate identity. They transform static belief into living movement, faith made visible.

2. Psychological Difference

In psychology, affirmations strengthen self-concept and reframe thought patterns. Declarations go further; they activate neural and behavioral alignment with purpose. By declaring action "I rest peacefully," "I forgive freely," you invite your body, mind, and spirit to cooperate in healing. The words become instruction, not just inspiration.

3. Spiritual Difference

Biblically, "I AM" is the name God revealed to Moses, the eternal identity of Being itself. When we declare, "I walk," "I speak," "I love," we move from reflection to co-creation. A declaration is faith spoken aloud in motion. It mirrors divine partnership: God is, and through His image in us, we become.

Summary Table

Aspect	"I Am" Affirmation	The Declaration Poem
Focus	Identity	Embodiment
Energy	Reflective	Prophetic
Voice	Self-definition	Faith-activation
Purpose	To believe	To live
Result	Reframes mindset	Reprograms movement

Conclusion

Affirmations remind us of our true selves. Declarations reveal how we live because of who we are. One is the seed of faith; the other, its harvest. Through the Declaration Poem, words become living actions, and faith becomes a daily rhythm of healing, peace, and purpose.

The Meaning of Glendina

Defined and Authored by Glendina Green © 2025 Global Creative Group LLc

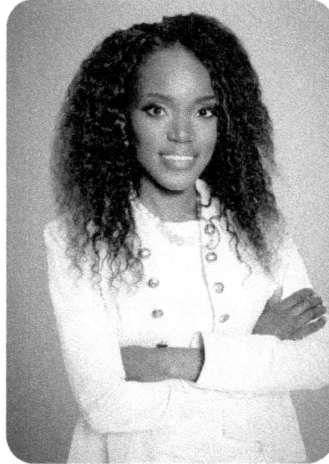

My decision to write about the meaning of my name stems from a lifelong curiosity. My parents never explained why they chose the name *Glendina,* and this absence of origin inspired me to assign meaning through personal reflection. In this season where the hero in me rises, I've chosen to give my name a voice, a purpose, and a definition that mirrors the woman I am and the woman I am becoming. In this transformative season of my life, defining my name is a declaration of identity and a commitment to purpose. This process symbolizes self-awareness and intentional living. Moreover, I

A Steadfast Heart A warrior's Journey Through Stage Ovarian Cancer encourage others to engage in similar reflection, examining the personal

significance of their names as shaped by their values, experiences, and belief systems.

The Origin and Revelation of My Name

God, the foundation and author of my being, is the One who ultimately defines who I am. Through His divine guidance, my life, purpose, and very name have found meaning and direction. From this foundation, my mother Linda Green gifted me with my name and seeds of wisdom, my mentor Ambassador Dr. Renee Knorr helped me discover the power of my voice and name, and my spiritual parents Pastor Philip and JoAnn Braziel's affirmation of my prophetic calling have each added layers of understanding to my identity. Together, God's foundation, their influence, and my own awakening have shaped the full meaning of who I am. Below is the living definition of my name as I have come to know it through the journey of faith, prophetic purpose, and divine revelation. Identity is the combination of qualities, experiences, and values that make a person unique. My Identity, therefore, defines who I am as an individual.

Name: Glendina

Pronunciation: /GLEN-dee-nuh/

Part of Speech: Proper Noun, Feminine Name

A Steadfast Heart A warrior's Journey Through Stage Ovarian Cancer
Origins: etymological, biblical, symbolic, and personal life

experience as defined by Glendina Green (United States, 2025)

The Meaning and Hidden Pattern of My Name

Etymological & Biblical Meaning

Glendina unites glen ("valley") and Dina (from Hebrew דִּ֫ינָה, Dinah, meaning "vindicated/judged righteously"). Together they form "Pure Valley of Vindication."

Green symbolizes renewal, growth, and life, the flourishing color of divine restoration and resurrection.

Combined Biblical Pattern:
"One who rises in purity from the valley, vindicated by divine justice, bringing life and renewal to others."

Scripture echoes this hidden code:
• Psalm 23 – "He restores my soul; He leads me beside still waters."
• Isaiah 61:3 – "To give them beauty for ashes… the garment of praise for the spirit of heaviness."
• Hosea 2:15 – "From the Valley of Achor a door of hope shall open."

This foundation reveals a divine pattern:

Even in low places, the faithful are lifted to restore others.

Spiritual and Prophetic Expression
Meaning:
"A steadfast warrior of fortitude, resilience, creativity, and faith-based purpose; one whose presence radiates power, patience, and divine love beyond physical stature."

125

Though small in frame, she carries the spirit of a giant. Her faith inspires nations, and her creative light builds bridges of healing and

understanding. She stands as a Global Influence Leader and Social Change Advocate, guided by a lifestyle rooted in love, compassion, and wisdom. Her voice moves hearts; her patience disarms storms; and her resilience transforms adversity into purpose.

Global Calling and Legacy

Her influence extends across the world, refining personal evolution through enlightenment, elevating it through inner renewal, and sanctifying it through faith in God. She is a living pattern of Isaiah 58:12 — "The restorer of paths to dwell in.

Symbolism and Hidden Attributes

Symbolic Element	Spiritual Meaning	Biblical Alignment
Strength in Gentleness	Power refined by peace	Matthew 5:5
Courage in Compassion	Boldness anchored in love	1 Corinthians 13:4–7
Light in Learning	Wisdom as illumination	Psalm 119:105
Healing Through Faith	Restoration through belief	James 5:15
Global Influence Through Purpose	Transforming nations through truth	Matthew 28:19
Abundance Through Divine Alignment	Prosperity as purpose fulfilled	Deuteronomy 8:18
Elevation Through Renewal	Rising through continual transformation	Romans 12:2

Personal Reflection
"My name is a covenant of calling every letter a testimony, every syllable a sound of renewal. In every valley, I find vindication; in every challenge, divine purpose. I am Glendina Green a steadfast warrior whose name sings the melody of grace, healing, and global transformation."

www.ingramcontent.com/pod-product-compliance
Lightning Source LLC
Chambersburg PA
CBHW081155270326
41930CB00014B/3162